D1527024

NOBODY HERE WILL HARM YOU

NOBODY HERE WILL HARM YOU

MASS MEDICAL EVACUATION FROM THE EASTERN ARCTIC, 1950–1965

BY SHAWN SELWAY

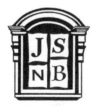

James Street North Books is an imprint of Wolsak and Wynn Publishers, Ltd.

Cover image: photographer unknown, courtesy of Gerda Selway (née Van Wanrooy)
Cover design: Marijke Friesen
Interior design: Julie McNeill, McNeill Design Arts
Author's photograph: Khantavy Sayavong
Typeset in Adobe Caslon
Printed by Ball Media, Brantford, Canada

The publisher gratefully acknowledges the support of the Canada Council for the Arts, the Ontario Arts Council and the Canada Book Fund.

 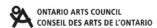

James Street North Books
280 James Street North
Hamilton, ON
Canada L8R 2L3

Library and Archives Canada Cataloguing in Publication

Selway, Shawn, 1948-, author
    Nobody here will harm you : mass medical evacuation from the eastern Arctic, 1950-1965 / Shawn Selway.

Includes bibliographical references and index.
ISBN 978-1-928088-09-7 (paperback)

    1. Inuit--Medical care--Canada--History--20th century.
2. Tuberculosis--Canada--History--20th century. 3. Inuit--Health and hygiene--Canada--History--20th century. I. Title.

RC314.S44 2016   362.19699'5008997124   C2015-905100-2

Perhaps you are wondering why you are brought down from your home leaving your friends and perhaps family behind. The reason is that you are sick, and if you were left at home, you may endanger those at home. So you are here to get well again. When you are well you will go home. We are all your friends here and want to try and help you get well. Things are strange to you, our food, our hospital and even our people look different to you. But do not be afraid. Nobody here will harm you.
 – *Mountain Views*, the newsletter of the Hamilton sanatorium, 1955

For in evils that cannot be removed without the manifest danger of greater to succeed in their rooms, wisdom, of necessity, must give place to necessity. All it can do in those cases is to devise how that which must be endured may be mitigated, and the inconveniences thereof countervailed as near as may be; that when the best things are not possible, the best may be made of those that are.
 – Richard Hooker, *Of the Laws of Ecclesiastical Polity*, Book 5

Le travail de l'historien, comme tout travail sur le passé, ne consiste jamais seulement à établir des faits, mais aussi à choisir certains d'entre eux comme étant plus saillants et plus significatifs que d'autres, à les mettre ensuite en relation entre eux; or ce travail de sélection et de combinaison est nécessairement orienté par la recherche, non de la vérité, mais du bien. L'opposition réelle ne sera donc pas entre l'absence ou la présence d'un but extérieur à la recherche même, mais entre des buts différents; non entre science et politique, mais entre une bonne et une mauvaise politique.
 – Tzvetan Todorov, *Les abus de la mémoire*

CONTENTS

PREFACE

Often when we propose to revisit the past in order to come to some reckoning with it, we are told that, even with perfectly complete information (obviously impossible to obtain), we cannot do so with an appraising eye, because *times have changed* and *today's standards* cannot be applied to the choices of those who went before. We cannot cast blame upon our forebears for doing what they thought was right, which we now think to be wrong, and, especially, we cannot exact a penalty from their inheritors in our day, in order to compensate the heirs of the wronged. We cannot punish the grandchildren for the sins of the fathers.

There is of course a danger that whenever we regard the past we will assume, from the supremely privileged place of hindsight, a moral superiority fraudulent because untried. What would we ourselves have done, had we been there, in the thick of things? In our own lives, don't we put ourselves first? Don't we look away and shirk responsibility? Catherine Merridale, in preparing to write *Night of Stone: Death and Memory in Twentieth-Century Russia*, spent two years after her archival research travelling among the Russians to speak with them about the past. She spent much time in the offices of Memorial and other organizations working against amnesias, official and not, and in the end warns that while she often felt at home in those places,

> there is also something darker going on. When you are incorporated into the society of these people, you are tacitly exonerated from complicity with the murderers and bureaucrats whom they have worked to expose. You are one of "us." The gnawing question, what would I have done, would my courage have failed, would I have colluded, is answered,

effortlessly. The nightmare is silent. You walk in at the end of the drama. You took no decisions, ran no risks, and still you get to share the flowers... The illusion is seductive, and it is deadly. It creates a fantasy world where ethical choices appear simple, where good and evil have been exposed, and where, by doing very little, anyone can feel they have joined the better side. Real life was not like that at any time. (Merridale, 345)

But it is not presumptuous to want to have the most complete conversation possible about the past and the present, and about how the past may bear on the present, precisely because we ourselves are now in the thick of things and having to make decisions in uncertainty. But to what extent is it possible? That depends on the extent to which there is a permanent human nature, in the sense of an endowment shared in by the members of each and every generation. I do not see how it can be denied that we are each of us endowed, in some measure, with a power of discrimination and a sense of proportion that allows us to reach just judgements by making and equilibrating many fine distinctions – more shades of green than we can put names to, more niceties of intention in a few moments of conversation than we could describe in less than twenty pages.

In judging the deeds of others, our contemporaries, we assume first of all the presence in each person of that power of discrimination and that sense of proportion, which we experience in ourselves, and, along with these, the capacity to recognize and in some measure oppose their circumstances, which we rarely take to be entirely compelling. This being so, it follows that if something is seen to be wrong now, it was wrong in the past also and would have been seen to be wrong. On the alternative, the inference must be that those who went before were either wicked – that is, knowingly did wrong – or unfree – that is, were somehow compelled (how is not clear) to act upon reasons we now consider delusion, or information that was incomplete. Moreover, we ourselves are similarly unfree, and perhaps similarly deluded as to our freedom. This seems to me initially plausible, but finally wrong.[1]

We recognize it can be difficult or impossible for us to learn enough about former circumstances to confidently evaluate their weight in past choices. Important details may be lost and forgotten altogether. Some experiential details may be quite unknown to us, or require a sharing in the experience that is no longer available. For example the "kayak-angst" used by Daniel Merkur in his interpretation of Inuit accounts of shamanism is not an easy experience to come by. Or consider the remarks of Viktor Shklovsky, who observed that Russian classicists enduring a lean post-revolutionary winter began to understand why fat is spoken of so frequently in the *Iliad*. And there are other, even more volatile or perishable circumstances also governing our choices. The general mood of the era, the common expectation, influences most of us by vaguely delimiting the horizon of the possible.

Even were we able to reconstruct all of the circumstances attending this or that choice in the past, there are other difficulties. The conception of responsibility varies in extent and character. It varies with the means available to address the circumstances, and also with one's understanding of who are one's own – that is to say, according to one's notion of those to whom it is permitted to do evil, and those to whom one is obliged to do good. In this regard, individuals do indeed stand to their opinions largely as inheritors, ignorant of the provenance of their own mentality. Largely, but not entirely. Truth is not only made, but found. There is a world that regulates our concepts, and that world includes what is permanently true of human beings, who show some regularities. But our freedom is elusive and intermittent, it flickers in the midst of miasmic unfreedom, of our often overwhelming urge to do and say just as others are doing and saying, even when there is no penalty attached to dissent. This is what lends plausibility to the relativist, historicist claim. But a few sometimes resist their fellows, the inertia of whose opinions is what is meant by *the times* in phrases like *the times have changed*. Some resist but most do not. This is an undeniable political fact. But it is senseless and slavish to maintain that whatever those who went before could not or would not resist, we too must accept and cannot resist. Nor would any reasonable person advance the corollary for the present that we should simply cease attempts to distinguish the better from the worse, and yield without resistance whenever we face pressure to act against what seems right or better to us. If, in looking back, we think we can discern how circumstances of whatever kind compelled a particular choice, and these circumstances are changed and no longer in force, then the choice can be remade – that is, its unfolding consequences arrested or undone.

More, if we have an unchanging nature, then now is to that extent perpetual and changeless and the distinction between now and then is rather weak. In that sense, there are no *times* that can change. Accordingly, if circumstances change, then remaking a choice or redressing a wrong is the just course, whether the initial choice was made last year or a hundred years ago. In the Canadian situation, the matter often takes the shape of a claim that the descendants of dispossessed persons are themselves in want or distress because of that earlier dispossession. More often still, what is sought is not only, or even, material compensation but rather acknowledgement that a wrong was done. From this acknowledgement can follow reconciliation, if it is desired, based on what has now become a joint interpretation of a mutual history. Or perhaps it would be better to say a revised official version of the history, established by the state with the issuing of an apology. It is unclear to me how much reconciliation can truly occur in consequence of an apology and a payment, delivered by the state, and costing me nothing whatever personally. Where is the atonement? Even a line item on the income tax form would have some meaning, though I suppose that there would be serious resistance to such a measure from all sides. Every month brings new reports of past abuses, but a real reckoning never seems to occur.

Of course, recognition of past wrongs does not guarantee the virtue or good behaviour of any party in the present. Revision can be abused, especially where reconciliation is not sought; but again, this cannot be a justification to abandon attempts. Ours has been a very dynamic country, and remains so in many respects. We are receptive to technical innovation and absorb large numbers of newcomers every year. But we are stalled on three enduring problems: how to reduce our burden on the land, how to replace the tacit accommodation of Quebec's particularity with an explicit agreement and how to undo the consequences of the crimes and errors of a settler state in order to allow full Aboriginal participation in Canada. The historical episode recounted here was not a crime, but it did involve some participants in error. Of course, there are Quebecois and Aboriginal persons who do not see the perfecting of the federation as a project worth doing. But I think it is, and accordingly what follows is offered as a contribution to the understanding of what previously was termed the *Indian Problem*, but that we now perceive to be the Aboriginal peoples' *Canadian Problem*.

INTRODUCTION

Mycobacterium tuberculosis, the agent of the disease in humans, is an ancient organism. Our species has been feeding and sheltering this microbe for a very long time, and it continues to cause a great deal of misery over large areas of the globe. When the lung is the affected organ, tuberculosis manifests itself to the sufferer as malaise and fever in the early days; then weight loss and persistent cough, with maybe a streak of blood in the phlegm from time to time; and then shortness of breath, and, if nothing else occurs (this is not usual; fungi and other opportunists generally become involved), there is a hemorrhage or two or three. Rarely, the person drowns immediately. Commonly, the flow is not enough even to interfere much with breathing, and after some minutes or hours, the blood thickens and the cough diminishes until it and the bleeding cease . . . until the next time. Maybe at the end there is the rupture of an aneurysm that has developed in a pulmonary artery owing to the fact that once-supportive tissue has disappeared, leaving the blood vessel hanging loose in a cavity. Otherwise, it is usual for the dying to fall silent before passing, so exhausted by spasm and blood loss that they are unable even to clear sputum from the larynx (Dormandy, 110).

Tincture of opium was the only real relief available, and was widely used in Europe and North America, where it helped hundreds of thousands of the afflicted to die in peace, and so greatly comforted those who held them in their arms (ibid., 49).

If the larynx itself becomes diseased, there is hoarseness and small ulcers. The contents of a tubercle may leak into the cerebrospinal fluid that bathes the brain and the spinal cord, and the resulting inflammation and swelling causes intense headache, chills, fever and drowsiness. The neck becomes stiff and bending the head forward causes great pain.

Without chemotherapy, "death supervenes," as clinicians phrase it, almost always. Most of the more superficial lymph nodes are in the head and neck region. Should these become tuberculous, they are apt to erupt through the skin, and the exposed sores intermittently exude a thick pus.

Then there is tuberculosis of the eyes, and tuberculosis of the bones and joints. In the latter, the spine, hip and knee are the most frequently affected, and children more commonly afflicted. Destruction of vertebrae and adjacent discs produces a humpback posture. Cavities in tuberculous bones or joints may eventually drain through fistulae that conduct purulent material to the surface of the body. A photograph of this development published in 1909 shows, for example, a young child facing a wall in order to expose for the photographer the back of their leg. The calf is splinted and bound. The back of the knee is swollen and discoloured, and several suppurating openings about the size of a fingertip can be seen in the flesh (McCuaig, 7).

The era of truly efficacious treatment of these atrocities dates from 1952 with the discovery of a cheap, orally administered chemical therapy for the disease.

> CASE 3 (K.R.) This 24-year-old Negro female was admitted to Sea View Hospital [Staten Island, NY] on November 7, 1951 . . . On admission . . . her status was critical. In the previous months her weight had decreased from a normal of 125 pounds to approximately 80 pounds . . . Therapy with Marsilid was begun on November 24, 1951, at 4 mg. per kg. per day. Within a few days the patient's temperature began to descend and reached normal in ten days. Two sputum examinations in the first two weeks of therapy were positive for acid-fast bacilli. However the following week . . . sputum was negative for tubercle bacilli and five subsequent consecutive examinations have been negative . . . The patient is continuing to receive therapy and is clinically completely asymptomatic, without cough or expectoration and with excellent appetite. She feels strong and is at normal weight. (Edward H. Robitzek

and Irving J. Selkoff, *American Review of Tuberculosis*, April 1952, quoted in Caldwell, 267)

Unlike earlier miracles, which had proven heartbreakingly deceptive, this one was real and lasting. It was also devastating for the institutions that had grown up around the disease.

The therapeutic labours of the preceding century had produced a program that amounted to a movement. Large fundraising and publicity apparatuses were in place, and the buildings they financed dotted the landscape of Western Europe and North America. Canada had beds for eighteen thousand (McCuaig, 282). There were four hundred seventy-one sanatoria in the United States alone. Within their walls anxious patients followed elaborate and punctilious routines, or underwent ever more drastic surgery. None of this was very successful. The death rate did fall from about 1900 on, but whether from improved sanitation due to urban reform, sanatorium segregation, both or neither is not clear (F. B. Smith, 240; Dormandy, 239). Through the 1940s in the US, twenty-five percent of all patients died while in hospital, and fifty percent of all released patients died within five years of discharge (Caldwell, 116). In the late forties, however, streptomycin and para-aminosalicylic were discovered, and combinations of them were devised that minimized both side effects (for example, inner ear damage, causing deafness or dizziness) and the production of resistant bacilli. Streptomycin turned out to be one of Nature's meaner jokes. After four weeks of treatment, drug resistant bacilli appeared. After sixteen, ninety percent of patients were producing the improved bugs. The more carefully investigators looked, the worse the news. In a foreglimpse of our current predicament, lab workers even found germs that preferred streptomycin to their normal food (Ryan, 328). However, in 1952 the excellent results of the American trials with isonicotinic acid hydrazide (INH) were published, and it soon became evident that this drug, used with streptomycin, was bactericidal, and the combination, truly wonder-working. Three months of treatment with them sufficed to eliminate infection from ninety percent of patients. In the fall of 1954 the sanatorium at Saranac Lake, a flagship of the American campaign since 1885, led the way again and shut down (Caldwell, 116).

With seven hundred fifty beds and a staff of four hundred eighty-four, the Mountain Sanatorium in Hamilton, ON, was, in 1950, the largest in the country.[2]

In addition to the fifteen buildings given over to patient accommodation and treatment, there was a central laundry, a radio studio and a farm, whose dairy operation eliminated the risk of tuberculosis from what up until 1914, when the state began to intrude upon milk production, was the second great reservoir of the disease. Extensive grounds ran up to the wooded edge of the escarpment, from where people strolling could admire the lake beyond the city below.

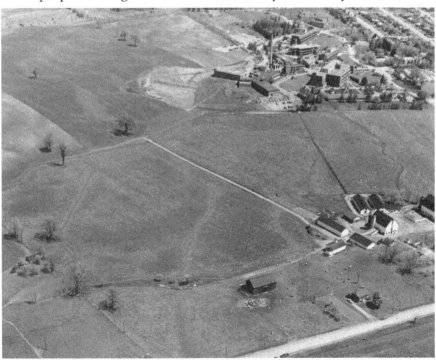

Aerial view of Hamilton's Mountain Sanatorium, 1968. Courtesy of the Archives of the Hamilton Health Sciences and the Faculty of Health Sciences, McMaster University, Hamilton Health Sciences Fonds, Hamilton Health Association Subfonds (hereafter Archives of HHS & FHS), 1980.1.73.7.22.

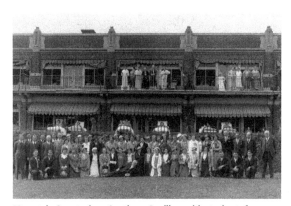

Mountain Sanatorium Southam Pavilion with students from Hamilton's Normal School on their annual visit in 1933.
Courtesy of the Archives of HHS & FHS, 1980.1.86.3.12.

By May 1952, one month after Robitzek and Selikoff published their results, twenty Hamilton patients were receiving INH. By January 1954, the first beneficiaries of the new therapy were already departing and the bed count was sinking rapidly, leaving the Hamilton Health Association (HHA), which managed the San, with an underused facility, a one-and-a-half-million-dollar building plan and a million-dollar bank account, all dedicated to the treatment of a vanishing disease.

But now patients from the North began to come in, at first Cree and Inuit from James Bay – seventeen in March, and fifty-one in October.[3] This anticipated a federal decision to concentrate Inuit medical evacuees in groups of fifty or more, in order to ensure them of companionship during periods of treatment that could continue for up to two years (Duffy, 72).

In November, Dr. Percy Elmer Moore, Director of the Indian and Northern Health Services branch of the Department of National Health and Welfare, was making arrangements for the Mountain Sanatorium to become the primary reception centre for Inuit hospitalized in Eastern Canada. Charles Camsell Hospital in Edmonton would perform similarly for the west. Five years later, readers of the HHA bulletin were informed that "in the past seven or eight years about a third of the Eskimo population of the Eastern Arctic passed through the Mountain Sanatorium . . . Now, however, this task in the battle against tuberculosis is being completed . . . This successful attack in [sic] T.B. among the Eskimos has probably saved the race from extinction."[4] Setting aside this particular claim, there is no doubt that aggressive measures taken from 1945 to 1960 had greatly reduced TB mortality in the Arctic (Wherrett, 117–18). These measures included extensive x-ray surveys for the disease and frequent evacuation for lengthy stays in southern Canada, since it was believed by doctors that treatment necessitated segregation and disciplined surveillance, and this entailed removing patients to a controlled, closed setting – quite apart from questions of costs, which in the North were almost double per capita what they were in southern Canada. According to R. Quinn Duffy, by the end of 1956 a thousand persons, representing ten percent of the total Canadian Inuit population, were in southern hospitals, most being treated for TB (71).

Suggestive as the numbers are for the importance of this episode for Inuit history, they also point to the great benefit derived by southern hospitals from the presence of these patients. Large contingents – up to three hundred concurrently – of Cree and Inuit evacuees, and the steady replacement of discharged Inuit by new admissions, greatly helped to stabilize the operations of the Hamilton Health Association during this critical period. In all, some 1,274 Inuit passed through and, thanks to the subsidy provided by their federal guardians, the hospital continued to run at capacity and show a surplus while its managers redefined its purposes.

Had these patients been asked, their likely preference for treatment nearer home might have yielded to considerations as to how this could practically occur, given the uncertainties of the current chemotherapies and the requirements of the doctors should surgery be necessary. But they were not asked. Nor was there at that time any means of broad consultation. Patients and their families did have a champion, self-appointed, in the person of the Right Reverend Donald Marsh, Anglican Bishop of the Arctic. The church had been trying for many years to get more hospitals built in the North, but could not obtain Ottawa's cooperation. The Anglicans had operated St. Luke's Mission Hospital in Pangnirtung since 1931. Beginning in 1951, Marsh advocated construction of a TB hospital in Iqaluit to serve the Eastern Arctic, with patients travelling by air. Moore rebuffed him on the grounds of efficiency.

By 1960 most surviving sanatoria were winding down, and thoracic surgery in the treatment of tuberculosis was nearly finished. The repercussions of evacuation and medical internment however continued. It was very difficult for men and women parted from dependents for whom they could do nothing to provide; and it was especially hard for those left behind if their near relations died in southern Canada, as little or no information about the death was given to those waiting back home. Although much had been done to mitigate the initial cruelties of the campaign, the anxiety and loneliness occasioned by sudden and prolonged separation reverberated for decades.

By 1963 almost all evacuees were back in the North, undergoing further experiences of centralization and schooling with their fellows, and by 1970, when the seven hundred camps of 1950 had become forty permanent settlements, it was clear to some that "welfare colonialism" was increasingly unworkable on all sides.

The medical evacuations were part of a larger set of interventions conceived as a new beginning in Euro-Canadian relations with the Aboriginal peoples in the North, and were carried through by sophisticated colonial administrators on behalf of a country that had become rather wealthy – certainly by comparison with pre-war circumstances – and of a state that was far more provident than ever before. To gain a sense of the enormous changes they wrought it is helpful to compare two medical cases for which we have solid information.

In 1931 Jennie Kanajuq succumbed to tuberculosis during an epidemic in the Coppermine district (now Kitikmeot region, NU). Between June 11 and August 9, 1930, nine young persons died at the settlement. Over the next four months, eleven adults followed them. The sole European doctor in the Central Arctic, Russell Martin, visited backcountry camps and, finding Kanajuq at Rymer Point on Victoria Island with tuberculosis of the spine, persuaded her to come in to a tent hospital he had set up at Coppermine (Kugluktuk). There she died sometime after March 1931 when Martin, his repeated requests for more help and specifically for a sun lamp (thought to be helpful against TB of the bones) ignored, flew out to make his case directly to bureaucrats in Ottawa. His position was terminated for lack of funds, and he returned to Scotland to do what he could against the disease in that country. At the time of her death, damaged vertebrae had deformed Kanajuq's posture, and a fistula had opened in her back from a lung, making it increasingly difficult for her to take in air in the usual way (Vanast, 93). She was predeceased by three of her four children.

Her parents had been close collaborators of Diamond Jenness, the far-travelling student of Aboriginal life, and in 1989 Jenness's son obtained for Kanajuq's son recordings of his mother's voice made in 1915. Walter Vanast comments: "In the second decade of this century, the nation was able to mount an expensive expedition to document in detail the terrain and habits of the 'newly discovered' Copper Inuit. In a pre-airplane era it had the wherewithal to send a wax recording machine to Coronation Gulf to record Jennie's voice. Sixteen years later, however, when arctic air travel had become commonplace, it found it impossible to send her a sun lamp for her tuberculosis" (98).

Thirty-five years after Jennie's death, when Gerda Van Wanrooy completed the Canadian portion of her nurses' training and came to the Holbrook Pavilion of the Mountain San in November 1957 she was put in charge, after a trial period, of a room of eight boys. Six were Inuit, one was a local white child and another was a young Japanese-Canadian. She herself was a "New Canadian," as the parlance then was, having emigrated with her family from Holland. In 1957 there were about four hundred patients at the San, of whom two hundred two were Inuit and other First Nations evacuees.[5]

One of Van Wanrooy's charges, Ham, was a boy of ten or twelve, whose patient card has survived. These were posted on the wall above the beds, and Ham's card outlines his slow return to health from October 6, 1957 – "Body cast, leg cast" – to July 7, 1958 – "spinal fusion" – on to November 2, 1959 – "Walk to bathroom" – and thence on November 25 to "remain in bed with cast on leg school in wheelchair." Finally, on February 12, 1960, he was ready "to walk with boots during day. To wear supporting cast on foot and leg during night."

In all, Ham's treatment extended over twenty-eight months, during which he received the attentions of nurses, doctors, physical therapists and an assortment of other technicians, not to mention dieticians, launderers, cooks and teachers.

Canada could and should have done more for Jennie Kanajuq. But generally, if one was Aboriginal, receiving prolonged attention from Euro-Canadians was far more likely to hurt than to help.

In 1907, Dr. Peter Bryce, in his capacity as chief medical officer to the Department of Indian Affairs, reported on the results of a questionnaire he had obtained from fifteen of the thirty-five schools to which he had circulated it. At first glance, it seemed that about a quarter of the fifteen hundred children who had passed through these places in the preceding fifteen years had died of tuberculosis. When Bryce looked further, and added in deaths occurring among pupils after they had gone home, the figure went to forty percent (Milloy, 91). Bryce proposed reforms. These were partially implemented, on paper. Conditions highly favourable to the spread of infectious disease continued. When Dr. F. A. Corbett repeated Bryce's survey by going personally through western schools in 1920 and 1922, he found children with suppurating ulcers at Old Sun's school on the Blackfoot Reserve (Siksika, AB) and at the Sarcee boarding school near Calgary. Of the thirty-three pupils at Sarcee, all but four were visibly tuberculous. And so on (ibid., 99).

As John Milloy and others have recounted in considerable detail, in propagating the residential system throughout the country, a rivalrous clerisy insisted on assuming obligations in loco parentis that they were not able to discharge, while Ottawa consistently failed to insist that they do so. Many thousands of children suffered from a complete withdrawal of affection; from cold, hunger and overwork; or died of contagious diseases contracted in crowded quarters in shoddy buildings. Yet it was hardly the case that the churches lacked for work to do within the precincts of their own culture. What was wanted however was "entire possession" of the human material whose moral and physical regeneration was to be wrought. The phrase appears in the Annual Report of the Department of Indian Affairs for 1890:

"It would be highly desirable, if it were practicable, to obtain entire possession of all Indian children after they attain to the age of seven or eight years, and keep them at schools . . . until they have had a thorough course of instruction" (quoted in Milloy, xii).

By 1950 the residential school system was at a dead end, but still operating, and even putting forth fresh shoots in the North. In 1948, a campaign by Neil Walker, an Albertan superintendent in Indian Affairs to eliminate residential schools in favour of day schools did not prevent the building of a new residential school in Hay River. And as late as August 1958 Peter Irniq (eventually the second Commissioner of Nunavut) was removed ("kidnapped" is his term) from Repulse Bay to Turquetil Hall in Chesterfield Inlet, four hundred kilometres south (Irniq, 19). Walker, like Bryce and others before him, was persuaded that residential school conditions were ideal for spreading tuberculosis and thought this should stop (Milloy, 262).[6]

If Aboriginal persons were neglected or abused, non-Aboriginal residents of the Great Dominion did not necessarily fare a great deal better when coming into contact with authority during the first eighty years of the federation. The Chinese who had been recruited to build the cross-country rail link were first taxed to handicap the growth of their community, and then excluded altogether. In 1914 the federal government issued a proclamation setting out its attitude to "persons in Canada of German or Austro-Hungarian descent." It followed up with the War Measures Act, under which an eventual 7,762 "enemy aliens" were interned as prisoners of war, usually because they were jobless. These men, who had been invited to emigrate, were forbidden to leave, and then incarcerated and put to work building roads mostly in the mountains (Kordan).

In 1922, there were sixty thousand Jews in Montreal, and a third of the children attending Protestant schools were Jewish. There were some Jewish teachers, but no Jew could be a principal, nor sit on the school board. Taxes were a recurrent point of debate, with Jewish tenants claiming that while the proprietor wrote the cheque, the tenant obviously footed the bill. In April 1931, by an act of the provincial legislature (an "Act respecting the education of certain children in Montreal and Outremont"), Jews living in Quebec finally gained the right to send their children to Protestant schools, but lost the right to establish a separate school system previously granted. The Act of 1931 essentially accommodated Jewish particularity within the Protestant schools by prohibiting segregation, excusing absences on thirteen Jewish holidays and forbidding discrimination against Jewish teachers in appointments or promotions. Representation on the school board had to wait until 1968 (Rosenberg).

During the Great Depression, as the economy shrank and the conditions of life worsened, federal and provincial governments continued to decline responsibility – unless individuals were so insolent as to complain, in which event the very rapid response often included deportation. Thus, a certain Sophie Sheinen, a Jew of Russian origin who immigrated to Canada in 1927, was arrested in Calgary and convicted of taking part in an unlawful assembly, that is, of protesting in public. After she had completed a six-month sentence in Fort Saskatchewan Gaol, Immigration wished to deport her to Russia. There were protests organized by the Canadian Labour Defense League, who also relayed Sheinen's letter of complaint about her treatment in prison (Roberts, 136). By the end of her term, she said, she had lost thirty-five pounds and was spitting blood, details that incline us to diagnose the obvious. The Department of Immigration and Colonization, however, thought, or claimed to think, that her medical troubles were fabricated to forestall deportation, and had a doctor pronounce her "fit for travel." (Not quite the same as *well.*) It is likely that Sheinen's tormentors were prevaricating, as this was their consistent, if unwritten, policy – a policy they were able to carry through, as Barbara Roberts has shown, in an atmosphere of parliamentary and judicial "incuria" for two decades prior to World War Two (197). Despite much controversy and protest, officials during this time (1930–35) managed to disencumber the nation of twenty-eight thousand assorted communists, immoralists, job seekers and "accompanying persons" (ibid., 38).

In short, the arbitrary exercise of near-absolute authority by a handful of persons, to the great detriment of many thousands of our forebears, Aboriginal or not, was ordinary as dirt.

What then had happened in the interval between 1931, when Jennie Kanajuq was left to die, and 1947, when forty-two people who had been x-rayed the year before by a medical team on the Hudson's Bay Company (HBC) supply ship *Nascopie* were flown out to hospital? (Grygier, 69). The nation had gotten big and rich and much more knowledgeable. We were more numerous and had benefitted greatly from immigration. There had been many medical advances and great improvements in transportation. But what was crucial for the North was a newfound political will – the prolonged attention to problems that comes only from the perception of a strong, usually material, interest. Kanajuq did not matter to anyone (other than Martin) who was in a position to do anything to help – or at least did not matter enough. Her situation was too remote and too difficult. Money and manpower are always competitive prizes, and the return was not judged to be worth the expenditure. Around 1945 the will to act in the North arose from the threatening prospect of American dominance in a region thought to contain large developable resources, and the embarrassment consequent on Canadian facilities coming under the critical eye of outsiders. New wealth allowed that will to be expressed, and new conceptions of Canadian nationhood informed the expressions.

The wealth was the result of wartime expedients employed to maximize the national product: direct public investment, much of it in manufacturing plant, and mostly spread over many operations.

From September 1939 through 1945, Ottawa put nine hundred million dollars into twenty-eight Crown corporations and other assets. At war's end much of this was sold cheaply to those who would agree to continue the operation and so maintain employment for at least five years (Eggleston). The maturing welfare state also benefitted directly from the war-surplus bounty. The Charles Camsell Indian Hospital, so important as a tuberculosis treatment centre in the west, was transferred directly to the Department of Health and Welfare from the Canadian Army Medical Corp by Order in Council (Charles Camsell History Committee). (The corp had it from the Americans, who had it, in embryonic form, from the Jesuits.) Demand, which had been severely curtailed and directed by controllers husbanding resources for the war effort and allocating quotas to targets, was freed to sustain what administrative fiat and government cash had brought into being. These measures worked very well.[7]

Support for industry was augmented with a raft of public works to be prepared and then funded as the need for employment might arise; these included the St. Lawrence Seaway and the TransCanada pipeline. Meanwhile great efforts were made to re-establish the conditions for balancing the North Atlantic triangle in the customary manner, by using the receipts from sales to Britain of wheat, newsprint, lumber and bacon to pay for imports from the States. Credit was extended to the UK and some large outright gifts were thrown in as well. However, the triangle kept collapsing, and repeated attempts to stabilize it failed. The damage overseas was too great and recovery too slow (Granatstein, *How Britain's Weakness Forced Canada into the Arms of the United States*).[8] Consequently, trade with the US predominated, and some in government, already uncomfortable with American encroachment in the Arctic, were visited anew by the old spectre, dependence. The enduring Canadian misery – of needing to be included in the councils of both Britain and the US, yet neither presumed upon nor integrated by either, while also wanting special dispensations from both – continued to generate fresh anxieties and embarrassments.[9]

In addition to the continuance of the traditional roles of government as aide to development and manager of trade and taxation, the state took on a new task, that of provider of social security, or cash, to individual citizens. This occurred in part because the distinction between public works and social welfare had come to be seen by the experts who were now advising the government as outmoded. Both were now understood as tending to the same effect: maintaining the all-important aggregate demand that had evaporated with such drastic consequences during the Great Depression (Owram, 307–8).

By the mid-fifties the Canadian economy had settled into a pattern centred on resource exports to the United States, imports of machinery and other capital goods from the US for purposes of extracting these resources, and a large amount of American direct investment in all industries. Military preparedness and industrial development were tightly braided, and something new came into the Canadian national experience: prolonged, limited war (in Korea) without sacrifice on the home front, waged by volunteers only.[10]

Some production was at the most advanced level. The CF-100 Canuck twin-jet, all-weather plane, designed to intercept bombers coming over the high northern horizon, was powered with engines developed and made in Canada. Testing and machining of these components was work of great precision and drew in contributions from producers of novel stainless steel and magnesium alloy castings, gears, bearings and blades (Eggleston, 65). Because bomber technology continued to develop rapidly, the North American line of defense had to be pushed to ever-higher latitudes. The Pinetree Line of radar stations, at the 50th parallel, was completed in 1954. It was immediately followed by the Mid-Canada Line of ninety-eight more radar stations at the 55th parallel, and then by another seventy-eight along the 70th. Costs for two of the three were shared between Canada and the US (Granatstein and Hillmer, 184).

All in all, postwar reconstruction turned out to mean income support payments (Family Allowance and much improved old age pensions to start), the St. Lawrence Seaway and rearmament; but also, a new strain of nationalism as the Canadian people stopped conflating liberal democratic institutions with Britishness and detached a civic nationalism from the chauvinism of the loyalist portion of the population.[11] And there was a renewed commitment to global humanism, resurrected from the ashes of the war and given doctrinal form by the United Nations in the thirty articles of the Universal Declaration of Human Rights (December 10, 1948).

Historically only nation states had guaranteed the rights of their nationals – and only for their nationals. When tested by refugees seeking asylum before the war, the nations had failed to recognize the human rights of the stateless. Within Canada, ethnically Japanese-Canadians and residents were evacuated for resettlement from the west coast toward the interior. This was not a handful of persons.

Twenty-two thousand were removed from British Columbia and their property seized and sold. By war's end, some who had elected for repatriation – that is, expulsion to Japan – were still awaiting departure. The government issued Orders in Council to confirm the deportations, but now there was broad resistance, and finally cabinet felt obliged to rescind the orders. However, Japanese-Canadians were still forbidden to return to the coast for another two years, and Parliament ratified this injustice by a large majority (Igartua, 37–38). Nonetheless, hope was strong and the idealist spirit expressed in the UN's declaration – coupled with optimism about technological progress, and an accumulation of new wealth in Canada and the US – inspired not only dreams of universal brotherhood but actual plans for the eradication of communicable diseases, poverty and dependency.

This strong improving spirit was present also among the civil servants who became occupied with the newly assumed northern problem – only, in the first place, these men and women were employees of the state, which had interests not always identical with those of the inhabitants of the country, and so was necessarily colonialist, try as they might to treat the region as a protectorate rather than an unlocked cupboard. In the second place, even with the best will in the world, uninvited meddling in the lives of others is perilous at any time and place.[12] However, there is no doubt that northerners were experiencing many difficulties for which assistance was welcome.[13] While a new abundance and security were enjoyed in much of southern Canada, life in the North remained precarious as ever.

Here is an example from the 1950 issue of the *Arctic Circular*, the newsletter of the Arctic Circle, a salon that had been meeting monthly in Ottawa since 1947. In the winter of 1948 an older Inuk named Ootogoocho was travelling and hunting in the Piling area on the south shore of Baffin Island. With him were his young wife, her two sons by a previous marriage, aged four and six, and a seventeen-year-old adopted daughter. During the summer Ootogoocho had cached some caribou, but when he returned to the area in the winter, he was unable to find the cache. As there was no other game to be had, the group ate their sled dogs and then some of their caribou-skin clothing. The four-year-old died, then the old man, then the seven-year-old. Too weak to walk, the women began using the bodies for food. Finally a search party from Igloojuak (Cape Thalbitzer, about one hundred forty kilometres northeast of Igloolik) found the camp. Neither woman was able even to speak, but both survived (Arctic Circle).

In February of 1949, a group of eight Creswell Bay (on Somerset Island, NU) people fell ill from botulism. David Koomayak (age fourteen) and a friend walked for help, were frostbitten and had to be evacuated from Fort Ross. Koomayak lost both feet. Subsequently his mother, along with "two older boys with tuberculosis and a baby with a stiff neck" were flown out. Twenty years later Koomayak was hunting on artificial legs. "Once a Fibreglass limb broke while he was chasing a wounded bear. But he made the kill. Shortly after, he changed to wooden substitutes which . . . stand up better in cold weather and need a minimum of adjustments."[14]

One final example will do to illustrate the extreme hardships that were a recurring feature of northern life at the time:

> In March [1953] word came in to Igloolik that seven hunters were missing, having been carried out to sea on a huge ice floe. They were without shelter, warmth or food (unless they had managed to kill a walrus). And the temperature had gone down to forty below with a thirty-mile wind.
>
> For nine long and bitter days there was no word of them... Then the hunters returned, all with frost-bitten faces, fingers and toes, and four of them with badly frozen hands and feet. They had caught one walrus, but it had frozen hard and made difficult eating. Two of the older men could not walk, and one of them, Shapungalok, was brought to the post by dog team . . . Another five days went by before the plane was able to get in from the south. Meanwhile the post manager succeeded in getting on the air with Dr. Judge at Pangnirtung, 575 miles way to the east, and received instructions for treating his gangrenous patient.[15]

In addition to enduring brutal trials like these, the Inuit were also living with a very onerous burden of disease. While on Eastern Arctic Patrol (EAP) aboard the HBC supply vessel *Nascopie* during August and September of 1945, Dr. Crewson, an ophthalmologist from the Hamilton branch of the Canadian National Institute for the Blind (CNIB) and his colleague A. H. Tweedle examined one hundred twelve Inuit and twenty-seven Euro-Canadians. Of the Inuit forty-seven were fitted with glasses on the spot; and twenty-one others were fitted with frames, the lenses to be sent in later. "It was observed," they reported, "that the men were generally interested in being able to hunt and the women to sew. Many of both sexes have learned to read syllabic and reading glasses were necessary for the older Eskimo."[16] Other doctors on this same patrol found fifteen certain cases of tuberculosis among one hundred forty-five persons seen, and suspected many more. Meanwhile Dr. R. C. Hastings, travelling with the *N.B. McLean* as it serviced aids to navigation in Hudson Bay, noted that of thirteen children born at Wolstenholme (near Ivujivik) during the previous year, only one remained alive at the time of his visit.[17] Tuberculosis was present but who knew in what quantity? Smallpox vaccination had been neglected, and the risk of a sudden and devastating outbreak was very high . . . Clearly something had to be done, and this turned out to be a greatly expanded annual medical patrol to start, and then large-scale evacuation.

ONE: THE RATIONALE

1.

Effective treatment, and therefore empty beds, was one of the conditions that made evacuation a possibility, although evacuation was occurring well before 1953, when the triple chemotherapy began to make the sanatoria obsolete. Also contributing were new diagnostic aids. The tuberculin skin test was a rapid means of ascertaining exposure to the disease. Along with advances in x-ray photography, it expedited decision making, especially after 1955, when x-ray film began to be developed on the spot in the North, rather than being sent south for processing. However it often remained difficult to be certain of the diagnosis. The only sure confirmation of tuberculosis was by swab and culture, and TB grows thirty times slower than other bacteria. Development of the optimum chemotherapy took many adjustments before doctors settled on combinations of streptomycin, para-aminosalicylic (PAS) and isonicotinic acid hydrazide (INH).

As Frank Ryan makes clear in his history of the arrival of these drugs, without the chemists and the companies who employed them, there would have been no breakthroughs in the treatment of tuberculosis. And given the enormity of the burden of that disease, only vast quantities of agents effective at very low doses, delivered cheaply, could have made any headway against it. Also important were the large numbers of patients gathered in sanatoria – that is, in well-controlled circumstances – and the large proportion of that population who were beyond all other help than the remedy whose value needed to be assessed. Any chance, however desperate, is worth taking when all other possibilities have been eliminated. Thus the first patient cured of tuberculosis meningitis by administration of streptomycin was a one-year-old who received injections directly through her skull to a cerebral sinus (Ryan, 239). The combination of researchers, pharmaceutical company labs, sanatorium labs and patient population in many stages of disease produced, in the five years after its first successes, twelve hundred papers on streptomycin (ibid., 283).

Successful anti-TB drugs were the product of a medico-industrial complex that had arisen since about 1860 on a base of synthetic dyestuffs and pharmaceuticals by developing "networks for the systematic production of novelty" (Pickstone, 133). Allied in this complex were industry, the academy, agencies of the state and overlapping civil institutions: hospitals, clinics and sanatoria. So rapid and vigorous was its growth that INH, for example, was simultaneously worked up by three separate teams of researchers operating independently of each other – and in secrecy. The secrecy was not primarily for purposes of patent protection, but to avoid arousing the deeply entrenched scepticism of veteran TB fighters, who were apt to construe any claim on behalf of a novel treatment as hyperbolic and self-promotional. Nothing could be discussed too widely in early stages for fear of provoking the hostility of the doctors, or of raising false hopes among patients. Even should the new agent prove effective, there was little chance that supplies of the test substance would be available for more than a miniscule fraction of those who might benefit. It was not the discovery of the substance, but the discovery of the means to mass-produce it that mattered.

Streptomycin was the quarry in an intense hunt organized by soil scientist Selman Waksman and conducted by Albert Schatz and others at Rutgers College of Agriculture in New Jersey. When Waksman, prodded by the announcement of penicillin, finally acted on several clues he had ignored due to a lack of medical knowledge, he quickly found actinomycin. Strongly antibacterial, it also proved too toxic for use. But the promise was immense and the way forward seemed clear. Operating in a small laboratory in a university however, Waksman was helpless to produce, analyze and test more than a small fraction of the possibly effective compounds. For this he required the services of a business like Merck and Company. Commitments of this sort were not easily obtained. In July 1944, Merck managers and chemists met with Waksman and two of his colleagues from the Mayo Clinic. Despite the extremely promising results of animal trials conducted by Mayo doctors William Feldman and Corwin Hinshaw, there was great reluctance to divert resources from the ongoing work on penicillin, which was also difficult to make in quantity. George Merck himself was brought in to make the decision that shortly had fifty Merck scientists involved with streptomycin. When the results of that effort began to come in, Merck topped himself by providing gratis a million dollars worth of the drug for testing (Ryan, 234).

PAS was the result of a deduction made by Jörgen Lehman on reading a paper about the effect of aspirin on the growth of tuberculosis bacilli in vitro. Having made the deduction based on the principle of competitive inhibition, Lehman was able to order up a variation on aspirin that, provided to the bacillus, would have the effect of breaking off a key in a lock. Manufacturing that key turned out to be vastly more difficult than designing it. The crucial factor was Lehman's link to the small Swedish pharmaceutical company Ferrosan, and the presence at Ferrosan of chemist Karl-Gustav Rosdahl, who was able to synthesize the compound when all others had failed (Ryan, 246). The first version of Rosdahl's process still took five steps to complete. Not until 1947 did his colleague Sven Carlsten devise the one-step method that made the drug available in the needed quantities at an easily affordable price (ibid., 291). The process was improved again the following year, and by 1964 production was at three million kilos annually, versus four hundred grams a month in 1944.

Isoniazid was similarly the result of an elaborate exercise carried through by chemists. In this case Robert Benisch, working at Bayer in 1941, cut a pentagonal molecule at each of its bonds, obtaining five different chains to which he attached side groups. From these manipulations came the winning combinations that proved effective against tuberculosis. Once in hand, PAS proved ten times more potent than streptomycin. INH turned out to be ten times stronger again than PAS.

It remained to evaluate the problem of possible emergent resistance, which had been so deflating following the initial fabulous success of streptomycin. Index Medicus, a comprehensive bibliographic reference to medical journal articles, lists more than seventy studies involving isoniazid between July and December 1952. The promise held good. Moreover INH was cheap, and unlike strep, which must be injected, it was given orally. Better still, and unlike PAS, it was palatable. The potential for this drug to become an instance of disruptive technology was large; it certainly promised to disrupt sanatoria, though with a rapidity that was not easily appreciated at the outset.

Strep use in Hamilton had begun in January 1947, when a full course cost a thousand dollars. Shortly it was found that dosages could be lowered, resulting in savings. In July of the following year, the Ontario government agreed to supply the antibiotic to all cases recommended by sanatorium doctors. The year after that, strep began to be coupled with PAS. INH came into the mix early in 1952.

On May 20, 1952, at a meeting of the board of the Hamilton Health Association (proprietor of the Mountain Sanatorium), Medical Superintendent Hugo Ewart and board chair Harry Thode responded to questions about the drug, which was much in the news. Thode said that INH was under study but that sanatorium staff was still not convinced of its usefulness. Ewart added that "the growth of resistance ordinarily expected as use continued had manifested itself from the beginning of the use of the new drug. We are now using the drug on twenty to twenty-five patients and the Merck Company is supplying enough for thirty more in order that we may study this resistance factor."[18]

Ten months later Ewart was still planning an expansion of the facility and proposed to hire more help for the San's school, which employed a dozen full-time teachers and eight or ten part-timers. But then the tide began to go out. The improving health of INH recipients, which had reinvigorated their interest in education, kept on improving and suddenly the patients were going home.

In September 1953, the "bed state" declined to seven hundred five, about fifty below capacity. However, "a group of Indians and Eskimoes [*sic*] is expected from James Bay at any time now. Unless there were unusual admissions of this nature it was expected that the bed state would remain low until the latter part of the year."[19]

By mid-June Dr. H. E. Peart, the assistant medical superintendent, was in Moosonee, apparently prospecting for patients, and the board devoted most of its meeting to a discussion of their plan to build a new one-hundred-fifty-bed infirmary at a cost of one and a half million dollars. If TB continued to decline, this facility could serve as a general hospital. In any event, it was necessary to modernize and be rid of the older buildings, just as the main boilers and the telephone system were being replaced.[20]

In September, the finance committee reported that even though a building had been closed, the reduction of costs had not kept pace with the reduction in patient numbers. However, because other sanatoria were in even more difficulty, the per diem grant rate had been raised for all, so that the Mountain San had actually met all current expenditures and added $146,000 to its investment fund that year.

In October, forty-two of forty-eight patients expected from Moose Factory were children, and a shipment of x-ray films from the Inuit survey had been received and were being examined. The slight revenue surplus was because of higher per diems paid by Indian Health Services and the department of veteran's affairs.

In January 1955, the board heard that twenty-four Inuit had arrived from Quebec, but that thirty additional children expected had been delayed by an outbreak of chicken pox. Some of the implications of the sudden influx of Inuit patients were becoming clear – among them, the fact that the expense would be greater to care for them, as they would have to be entirely cured before they could be sent back to the rigours of life in the North.

Still, things were turning around. In February, G. B. Elwin reported for the finance committee that a maintenance profit of $10,800 had been realized for the month of January – largely due to the presence of many Aboriginals. Total occupied beds: seven hundred fifty-five, near capacity. In April, the board learned that a saturation survey of the south Baffin shore would be conducted, beginning in June. Two pictures were to be taken, one being developed on the spot and the other sent out with the patient if tuberculosis were diagnosed. This new method of surveying would allow suspected cases to be evacuated at once. The exodus of local patients continued. In June there were one hundred empty beds. However, the Inuit were expected to arrive shortly.

And indeed, by mid-October the monthly patient count averaged six hundred eighty-six, of whom nearly three hundred were Aboriginal. There were now one hundred fifty children in residence, and the nursing staff had been increased by five. The actual bed state as of October 18 was seven hundred twenty-eight. To sum up, from the inception of INH trials in May 1952 to October 1955, that is, in about three and a half years, the Inuit patient population grew from nothing to about three hundred. (Overall, there were five thousand people hospitalized for TB treatment in Ontario.) In 1956 the number rose to three hundred thirty-two, in a total of 1,578 Inuit undergoing treatment at all locations (Grygier, xxi). These patients had been diagnosed, sequestered and moved thousands of kilometres to be resettled in sedentary long-term accommodation – a considerable feat.

2.

Once the Canadian state accepted responsibility for Inuit health and therefore the high rate of TB morbidity, it remained to be seen who exactly would be selected to discharge that responsibility. As it happened, a group of mostly medical people, eventually operating within the Department of Health and Welfare, got the job. The details of how they obtained this authority are in the archives and have been studied by P. G. Nixon. What we would like to know is why the choice was made to evacuate about a thousand people a year, rather than treating these people in the North. Who actually made the decision, and on what rationale; and why was it done so poorly at the outset?

Nixon's research showed him that

a significant debate occurred within the federal public service during the late forties and early fifties over the appropriateness of applying a "western" model of medicine on northern natives . . .

With respect to the federal government's Inuit anti-TB campaign this paper will [argue] that the often nightmarish developments in this area are understandable not only in terms of a colonial political economy or the problems of cultural ethnocentrism and arrogance, but also because of: the logistics of program delivery in the particular area being served [and other political / bureaucratic factors] . . .

Such an analysis might allow us to say . . . that sanatoria treatment was chosen over domiciliary care because of the particular characteristics of this disease and for pragmatic administrative considerations, rather than because such treatment was the "culturally accepted form." And that people were wisked away without adequate notice to their families because of the naval method of transportation chosen for program delivery and the resulting requirements (because of ice and other weather-related factors) to enter and exit isolated communities often in a matter of hours, rather than evidence of disregard for the needs of a differentiated other. ("Early Administrative Developments in Fighting Tuberculosis among Canadian Inuit," 69–70)

Nixon establishes, from the record, the main point: namely that physicians were in charge, and that it was they who resisted proposals for northern treatment. Even the establishment of northern rehabilitation facilities that would permit the earlier return of evacuees was not liked. There was an opinion in Health and Welfare that no Inuit who had undergone major surgery or been in lengthy treatment in southern Canada should go back to the North (ibid., 79). Equally bizarre was the official assertion, reported by Health and Welfare Minister Paul

Martin to the prime minister, that his officials believed "once you move an Eskimo from his native environment to a hospital bed, the change is absolute and the location of the bed makes little difference. If the hospital bed is to be located at a distance greater than can be travelled by dog team, a few extra hours in an aircraft cannot make much difference to the patient, or to his family as regards visits" (quoted in Nixon, "Early Administrative Developments," 83–84). Apart from the fact that in this period we are talking not only of aircraft, the principal means of evacuation from the Western Arctic, but also of some weeks on a ship for those going south from the Eastern Arctic, the notion that latitude means nothing is preposterous. The mean July temperature in Hamilton is not that of Iqaluit. But why were the doctors so obdurate, why so strongly committed to evacuation?

What Pat Grygier found in the archives was that

> the arguments usually put forward for refusing to provide sanatoria treatment in the North were, first, that it is not possible to attract specialists to the region and that adequate modern treatment was therefore not possible; second, that the number of active TB cases was expected to decline within five years, so extra beds in the North would then be superfluous; and, third, that the main purpose of hospitalization in the North was not so much to give active treatment as to remove the infection source from the community, which could be done using the present facilities. (73)

This last, removal, had been ordered by P. E. Moore, the official in charge of the branch of Northern Health and Welfare dealing with Inuit and First Nations health. Doomed individuals were to stay in the North; the treatable were to come out.

The principal argument, however, seems to have been cost. Hospitalization was simply cheaper by almost half in southern Canada. Cost aside, was treatment in the North a practicable, real option, given the state of medical knowledge about the existing therapies? Moore thought not:

Irrespective of expense, someone else will have to demonstrate that it is possible to retain first rate chest surgery teams, operating room nurses, laboratory facilities and blood banks in the far north. We and Bishop Marsh know too well the problem of recruiting and retaining general duty doctors and nurses for isolated communities to say nothing of the highly skilled specialists who must have a constant volume of their special work in order to retain skill and judgment. And who is going to maintain these elaborate institutions when we either get tuberculosis under control or in failing, lose the population they were intended to serve?[21]

And then, what is the point of trying to weigh the question, why does it matter? It seems that discussion is foreclosed by unanimous agreement on the intensity of the danger posed by the epidemic to the whole people. At the same time, the manner in which the something was done is much faulted. First there is a vague and never argued notion that more treatment could have been carried out in the North. Second, there is a conviction that the abrupt and cavalier way in which evacuation was done was wrong. These are two quite different questions.

3.

The big breakthrough with isoniazid did not occur until the fall of 1951, and the drug was still in limited use by the spring of 1952. It is important to note that the evacuation policy preceded the great emptying of the beds in southern Canada. In June 1953, while there were only eight Inuit recorded as patients at the Mountain San, one hundred thirty were already resident at Charles Camsell Indian Hospital in Edmonton, and one hundred two were at Parc Savard hospital in Quebec City (Grygier, 77). These were the principal centres in the west and east. The Charles Camsell had begun as a Jesuit College in 1913, served as a base for the US army during the construction of the Alaska Highway, had been renovated by the Canadian military after 1944 before passing to Health and Welfare and opening, in 1946, as a TB sanatorium. (Parc Savard had been the Quebec Immigration and Detention Hospital before the campaign against TB in the North began to take on serious momentum in 1950.) In short, evacuation was preferred from the outset of that campaign, at a time when beds were not waiting empty but had to be acquired. In eastern Canada, however, the advent of isoniazid resulted in a shift of patients from Quebec and James Bay to Hamilton.

Beginnings are difficult. Early chemotherapy of TB had a bitterly deceptive development, complicated by uncertainties about preventive vaccination. Bacille Calmette-Guérin (BCG) promised to block the multiplication of the bacilli in the infancy of its human hosts, and was favoured in Canada, but not in the United States.[22] Two drugs were in use prior to 1952. Streptomycin had been available since 1947. After 1948 it was given in combination with PAS. These drugs were effective, but tremendous uncertainty remained about the long-term consequences of their use. Indeed, by 1952, large studies conducted in Britain and the US concluded that about twenty percent of pulmonary infections were not touched by the drugs. The breeding of resistant strains continued to be the major worry, and it seemed inevitable that a bacillus resistant to both drugs would develop (Ryan, 341). There were also troublesome day-to-day problems with their administration, and lurking dangers of toxicity. Dosages were continually being adjusted, and there may also have been questions of racially specific responses, as well as the differences between adults and children.[23]

In 1960, A. R. Armstrong, Director of Laboratories at Mountain Sanatorium, was involved in sorting out the implications of a strong difference between Inuit metabolism of isoniazid and that of other recipients. At the time it was thought that forty-four percent of Caucasian patients were so-called rapid inactivators of the drug, versus a much higher proportion of Inuit. Metabolic destruction of the molecule in the liver made it unavailable to attack the tuberculosis microbe, although the problem was more complicated than that. Inactivation was owed, as we now know, to the presence of a liver enzyme that varies from race to race. The difference gave rise to the time-concentration problem: how much of the drug had to remain in the system for how long in order to inhibit the bacillus? Could it be that the Inuit who had been treated at the San had not been receiving the optimum dose? A review showed that the outcome of the standard treatment was the same for Inuit as for others (Armstrong, 16–17). On the other hand, it also seemed that the usual doses were bacteriostatic – that is, halted the growth of the bacillus, but not bactericidal. To kill the microbe outright, higher doses were needed.

Fifteen years later, the time-concentration problem returned in an entirely different context. Outpatient drug therapy or domiciliary care can be difficult to carry through because patients tend to skip doses or visits. Fully supervised therapy, however, is onerous for all if the patient has to come in frequently. Once a week is good, but then fast inactivators will derive less benefit from the same dose, and upping the dose will not help. If the extra is not toxic, it will be excreted or metabolized. But upwards of sixty percent of Inuit are fast inactivators, so researchers attempted to find a matrix therapy; a compound of isoniazid and a carrier that would be more slowly absorbed from the gut.

It is notorious among practitioners of any art or craft (as opposed to their managers and critics) that things frequently do not work as they are supposed to. The magic of technology is often offset by its unreliability. This sense of contingency, of the uncertain reliability of equipment and procedures would be coupled, in the case of physicians, with the experience of the idiosyncratic nature of patient response to treatment – not to mention the variation of nurse and physician response to education and experience. Not all medical professionals are or could be good at all things and medical attention must be continuously variable, treatment closely managed. It is not a matter of applying a remedy and awaiting the inevitable. In 2004, a vice-president of pharmaceutical manufacturer GlaxoSmithKline asserted that ninety percent of drugs are effective in only thirty to fifty percent of their recipients (quoted in Godfrey, 14–16).[24] There is also the matter of patient non-compliance, which can induce a strong medical preference for controlled circumstances around treatment.

Of greatest concern was the possibility of drug-resistant strains. This would have been a very great difficulty had it occurred in the North, because of the conditions of life and the comparative paucity of medical personnel. This danger in itself would have weighted the decision heavily toward evacuation. This choice offered at least the separation of the infectious from their intimates, with the additional possibility (unspoken, of course) of complete quarantine should a novel bug appear on the southern wards – where careful segregation by age, gender and degree of active disease was imposed. And of course there is always the other side of the coin – fewer controls in the North might have facilitated the spread of a new strain that could then come south. From this perspective, the evacuations were a police action in support of an undeclared quarantine. It would be helpful to know whether the few patients who were allowed to remain in northern (mission station) hospitals received the same drugs as those who were brought out.

Streptomycin was given by intramuscular injection. The dosage was varied not only for children but adults over fifty-five. Allergic reactions (fever, rash) occurred in some instances, though in less than ten percent of patients, as well as vertigo and visual difficulty. In 1953 doctors in Hamilton were trying a combination of streptomycin and dihydrostreptomycin.[25] Ten years later the latter, once preferred as causing less vestibular disturbance (vertigo), had been rejected as causing more deafness and was no longer used with children (Pagel et al.; Miller, Seal and Taylor). Injections were given daily, deep into the buttock or the outer side of the thigh, alternating between legs. Some patients felt pain directly after the injection, others later. The injections continued day after day, week after week, requiring skilful hands, sharp and sterile equipment, and no mistakes or tardily observed infections, allergic reactions or side effects.

PAS was taken orally, one to four times a day, in flavoured water. Most patients initially experienced flatulence and loose bowels, and some were nauseated. Hypersensitivity sometimes occurred in the second or third weeks, with rash and fever. Few children experienced these problems, but adults left to take PAS on their own would often quit.

Doctors at the Toronto Free Hospital for Consumptive Poor (more commonly known as the Weston Sanatorium) began studying the combination of strep and PAS in March 1948 and found that while there was no appreciable therapeutic advantage over strep alone, the combination greatly reduced incidence of completely resistant bacilli. Resistance was defined by culling bacilli from patients at monthly intervals before, during and for six months after treatment, then cultivating them and depositing a cross-section of the cultivar into petri dishes containing five different concentrations of streptomycin. The growths, if any, were compared to that on a control plate. When growth in the dish containing the highest concentration of strep was found, at the end of a month, to rival the luxuriance of that on the control plate, complete streptomycin resistance was said to have developed. (Presumably because the amount of strep required to kill that bug, if it were still killable, would have been too toxic for the human organism to withstand.) Although treatment shifted after the introduction of isoniazid toward a combination of that drug (also orally administered) and PAS, at Mountain San in 1953 – that is, immediately after the first successes of isoniazid – the standard chemo course was still strep and PAS, continued for a year or more. Nor did the introduction of INH ease uncertainty much at first. Some cases of peripheral neuritis were caused by the drug, experienced as a burning sensation in the skin of the arms and legs. These drugs were unpleasant to receive, and had to be taken regularly (and except for strep, daily), without interruption, except in the case of a bad reaction, when they were stopped, thus increasing the risk of emergent strains.

These considerations alone would likely have tipped the balance toward evacuation. To them were added several others. One was the unpredictable need for surgical follow-up to successful drug treatment. Typically this was done for lung disease that produced irreversible tuberculous foci, regions of tissue that were either dead or so dense that blood-borne chemicals could not reach them. Instances of bone disease might also require surgery, and surgery implies the availability of transfusion blood. A mainstay of treatment throughout the period however remained bedrest and nourishment, and any regimen was more likely to be maintained in a situation affording close supervision by large numbers of staff.

In addition to the doctors, nurses, clergy and teachers in attendance on the patients, many laboratory services were required.

The logistics of recruiting, transporting and supplying such an establishment for years at a time, even without the complications of the many tricky details of a still incompletely understood or routinized chemotherapy, would have dictated that the patients come to the services rather than vice versa. How much those in charge knew the extent of the interruption that evacuation inflicted on the lives of patients and of those left behind seems not to be known. It is disquieting, in view of the still-emphasized importance of the individual's mental state for their battle with the disease, that the rule was apparently waived for the Inuit – waived or trumped by the imperative to contain the disease – or perhaps seen as obsolescent after it became clear that a few months of chemo could do what years of rest previously could not. It is impossible to see how being sequestered on a hospital ship and transported to an unknown region of alien climate, vegetation and landforms, while leaving parents and dependents behind could have been anything other than extremely distressing. Indeed the contradictions were discussed within the circle of those on the front lines.

The inference is firstly that the doctors had changed their faith, without publicizing the fact. A long-held item of dogma – the efficacy of the rest cure – was being proven false. Sanatorium care under optimum conditions had really achieved little of physiological significance (hence the steady increase in ever more drastic surgery). The new drugs worked, and comparatively quickly; the personnel able to administer them and monitor their effects were on hand in southern Canada; and the sooner the ill individual could be brought in and cured, the sooner the danger for all would be reduced. Secondly, the epidemic was, for a time, construed as a state of emergency – the favoured circumstance of those holding power, since it is the easiest in which to act, the most broadly permissive. The complexities and inconveniences of distinguishing and negotiating a just course are all postponed for the duration of an emergency, when survival warrants rapid and drastic measures and enforced compliance. That said, the emergency period was short, a few years only, just before and after 1955 when two hundred persons were brought out by the EAP alone. It is bitter nonetheless to contemplate the contrast that existed after 1953 or so between the circumstance of the Inuit and those of their caregivers. Nurses and others at Mountain San were very happy in their work, which paid comparatively well. They lived in dormitories on site, enjoyed the egalitarian atmosphere and passed there some of the best years of their lives. For the Inuit it was a different story. They were grateful for the treatments that cured them, and averted the crippled invalidism that could have been their lot, or the death that was the fate of only twenty-seven of the twelve hundred or so Inuit who passed through the Hamilton San, but the price was high.

At present, the nurses involved describe the evacuations as high-handed and hurtful, but still conclude that lives were saved and a people brought back from the verge of extinction. They say that it was wrong to bring people so abruptly into such unfamiliar circumstances (food, climate, et cetera), and especially to accustom small children to one way of life in southern Canada and then return them to conditions for which they were entirely unprepared, with relatives who were strangers.

The full extent of Inuit discomfiture is not known. To my knowledge, we have only a few brief narratives of the sanatorium experience from the patient side.

Between 2007 and 2009 Emily Cowall conducted anthropological fieldwork in Pangnirtung, whose residents she had come to know during earlier work. Her project centred on patient photographs found in the Archives of the Hamilton Health Sciences and the Faculty of Health Sciences at McMaster University, which holds the records of the Hamilton sanatorium. The community, among which are several former San patients, identified the persons shown in the photographs and spoke about their time in the sanatorium. Cowall was hopeful that this would lead to an oral history of the episode: "However, as the project continued, the participants decided against sharing personal histories because they considered them to be private and not appropriate for a dissertation. They simply wanted to name their family members and receive copies of the photographs. Respecting their wishes, we continued the project, named individuals in the photographs, and celebrated the return of copies of photographs to the individual or their relative. I made the commitment to protect their privacy and respect the confidential information I heard and witnessed" (13–14).

Cowall does not explain why this decision was taken, or even if she was given any reasons, nor does she say if she has any notes and if so, where they are and if there is any set of circumstances under which they might become available to historiography.

The Qikiqtani Truth Commission, conceived in 2007 as an Inuit-led inquiry into sled-dog killings during the sixties, expanded its mandate to receive testimony about all aspects of the Inuit experience of the move into larger, permanent settlements. Medical evacuation to southern Canada and its consequences was often touched on by those who testified. It is disquieting to read in the commission's reports that its visits to the villages of Qikiqtani were the first opportunity that many individuals had taken to speak openly about their experiences, since the implication is that the Inuit record may still be sparse and in many cases uncollected.

Inuit accounts take the form of a captivity narrative. That patients were anxious and homesick could be observed or intuited by anyone, but cosmological unease, if the expression may be permitted, is not so readily discernible. There was some continuity for religiously observant Christian Inuit – almost everybody, it seems – in the ministrations of the Anglican Church. In addition to the sanatorium chaplain, who was always near (the Catholics, Jews and others were also served by their own clergy), Bishop Marsh, an Inuktitut speaker, visited when he could. (There was also Gladys McAndrew, a very faithful visitor to the wards, who was called upon in 1949 to look in on three Cree and one Inuit woman who had lately arrived at the San. For the next twelve years she went at least twice a week, and also attended at the train station or the airport when patients headed home.) Certainly at the time detailed knowledge of Inuit traditions was held by very few. Deprival in the matter of food was more important than questions of taste alone, but, for example, the importance of seal blood for the right composition of Inuit blood is not easily grasped; nor, to take another example, is the system of name-souls. Inuit children are named after one or another recently deceased relative until the relative is recognized and the name takes. Presumably infants born in the San could be named, because the mother would have still been home during much of the pregnancy and so have known who had died recently. But what was done in the North, if someone went south and no more was heard of them? What became of that soul or name? To examine these matters would take us too far afield, but I raise them in hope of conveying some sense of the scope of what is being left out when an account is restricted, as this one is, mainly to the Euro-Canadian side of things.

4.

In the final chapter of her study, Pat Grygier offers an eight-point indictment of the Canadian government's action or inaction on health care in the North.[26] The eighth point is

> the refusal of [Health and Welfare] to develop hospital treatment in the North, despite the presence of the mission hospitals and some mining company and American military hospitals already operating there. . . . Of course conditions were very difficult in the Arctic . . .
>
> But the mere fact that the handling of the programs improved in the late 1950s and 1960s without any change in the Arctic weather and geography – and with minimal increase, if any, of the technical development available – underlines the hollowness of this excuse. Military and mining operations, including some medical facilities, had been successfully established in many places by the 1950s. When the will and

money were there, the difficulties could certainly be overcome. (Grygier, 176–77)

(This overlooks the fact that the large military bases were paid for by the US, not Canada. The Charles Camsell and Clearwater Lake Hospital in The Pas, Manitoba, were also built by the Americans.)

It certainly is the case that the handling of the programs was improvable without "technical development" because what was missing was not equipment but personnel and only personnel – people assigned the responsibility of looking out for the mental comfort of the interrupted and dislocated evacuees, and of those they were leaving behind. But it is wrong to discount technical development, although it was more important earlier in the period than later. Technical advance around 1950, in particular the movement of war-surplus portable x-ray machines, and the use of the ship-borne helicopter, were important in making the anti-TB campaign feasible in the first place. But there was also a steady increase in the recourse to air travel in all seasons. And the art and science of medicine in 1960 was quite different than it had been in 1950. Again, this is a question that is susceptible to empirical verification – if one had access to the records, which remain confidential.[27] One could work through the nature of the treatment given, the length of the patient's stay in hospital, the number of pints of blood required and so on, case by case, and thus arrive at a plausible verdict on whether that patient could have been properly cared for in the North – assuming, always, that they would have accepted treatment in the first place, which is no small assumption. Unfortunately, we seem not to have full records but only discharge sheets for the Mountain San. Records do exist for Mountain's Toronto counterpart, Weston Sanatorium. Those for the years after 1960 are maintained at Weston's current successor, West Park Healthcare Centre, as active clinical records; those for the years prior to 1960, comprising some seven hundred fifty boxes, are in deep storage. But it was not until 1962 that Inuit were concentrated at Weston, and by then the deficiencies noted by Grygier and others had been remedied, and anyway outpatient chemotherapy was rapidly being implemented on all fronts, north and south, and was soon to replace hospitalization altogether as the standard of care.

There is another possible source of information: the records of St. Luke's Hospital in Pangnirtung, which have been investigated by Emily Cowall. She reports that

> in keeping with the Government's use of the Mountain Sanatorium, a record of patients diagnosed with tuberculosis appears in St. Luke's day books (as of September 1953) and was maintained until the hospital closed in 1972. Unfortunately, the day books do not reveal the reason why some were selected to stay in St. Luke's and why others were sent to sanatoria. Some insight into this process is contained in a letter from St. Luke's Head Nurse, Prudence Hockin, to Bishop Marsh on September 17, 1959. Hockin reports that the *C.D. Howe* arrived on 10 September, 1959 and departed for Hamilton two days later. She names six additional Inuit who were taken south, including a sixty-six-year-old male, a fifteen-year-old male, a six-year-old female from Pangnirtung (for the investigation of a kidney lesion), a twelve-year-old female from Pangnirtung (with an old injury of her knee), and a thirty-six-year-old male (for a hernia operation). Hockin (1959) adds, "They have evacuated the cases they found [of tuberculosis] but left the 5 we have here". I investigated Hockin's account with one of the individuals named in this letter, and she confirmed that she was not admitted to the hospital; instead, she recalls being taken to the ship and not being allowed to leave after her assessment. (insertion in original; 109)

This was late in the campaign, and by 1959 the southern medical team may have been more comfortable leaving people in the North than they had been earlier. However, this report does suggest that it was potential surgical cases that were being taken out. It also suggests that a comparison could be made of the treatments given at St. Luke's from 1945 or so with those available in southern Canada, which would help in assessing the necessity of evacuation in the earlier period. However, this would leave aside the question of capacity, which would always be susceptible to sudden spikes in demand. In the fall of 1941 the inhabitants of the Cumberland Sound area served by St. Luke's experienced three overlapping epidemics: paratyphoid (a bacterial infection), influenza and chicken pox. Apart from the increased load on the medical staff and their help, the inpatient count went from one hundred sixty-two in 1940 to two hundred eighty-eight in 1941, with all of the increase after August (Cowall, 70).

Another advocate for northern hospitalization, and one who knew firsthand its problems, was Dorothy Knight, the nurse at Lake Harbour (now Kimmirut) on the southern end of Baffin Island from 1957 to 1958. Knight went in on the *Howe* in the summer of 1957 – not very smoothly. Ice kept the ship off, then a measles case on board forced the medical officer to embargo all comings and goings. Finally she was helicoptered in, arriving in August, after a two-month journey from Montreal. In the afternotes to her as-told-to biography by Betty Lee about a year of anxious improvisation, Knight cannot quite reconcile herself to the evacuations.

> Was it absolutely necessary to take sick Eskimos away from their homes and families for years at a time? ... Later, I worked in Africa where the natives lived much as the Inuit did as far as inadequate housing and sanitation were concerned. But they were treated at home. It was found that hospitalization made little difference to the cure rate and that one need not remove the average TB case from his home to protect his family, because most household contacts had been infected by the time the cases were diagnosed, anyway ... One person in each village accepted the job of seeing that the TB patients and suspects took their pills. These pills contained drugs found to be effective against tuberculosis in the early fifties. (quoted in Lee, 235)

This last is ingenuous – there was great uncertainty in the early fifties about outcomes; confidence came with experience. The African comparison (Knight was in Lesotho) is feeble. Treatment "in their homes" implies a degree of concentrated settlement that was not usual in the Canadian Arctic – something that Knight actually described: she visited camps at considerable distance from her home base, and fretted because people did not seek her medical help. It is interesting that two of her three positive suggestions are technical: that camps be given radio equipment to communicate with the nearest nursing station, and microscopes be provided so that active TB can be detected by sputum examination. (The third thing she urges is of course training for Inuit health workers, so they can replace the Euro-Canadians in that role.)

As it happens, there is a much better and exactly contemporaneous parallel to our subject, and one that affords instructive comparisons. During its development, three independent sets of isoniazid trials were carried out simultaneously. One of these was led by Walsh McDermott at New York Hospital. McDermott was intimately acquainted with the disease he studied. He had begun his personal struggle with it in 1935, while training at New York. He went to Saranac Lake for treatment, then back to training. Over nineteen years he was hospitalized nine times and lost most of his left lung to the surgeons. It ended with isoniazid, which he began to study in 1949 after being sent to Europe to look into the German thiosemicarbazone program. By the end of 1951, the two American groups working on INH had a very promising drug and no further way forward for trials. "Studies with sulfa drugs and streptomycin had shown that pulmonary tuberculosis was a poor model for clinical research: its course varied from patient to patient, and its clinical criteria, especially chest X-rays, were [subjective]. To generate useful data in pulmonary TB, researchers needed to use the 'chance selection' method to compare new drugs to the existing standard, streptomycin. This new technique had recently demonstrated its power in the British Medical Research Council's randomized clinical trial of streptomycin for pulmonary tuberculosis. McDermott believed that two other forms of the disease, miliary (infection of the blood) and meningeal (infection of the central nervous system), provided simpler research models" (Jones, 62).

The course of miliary disease was entirely regular, predictable and fatal, and therefore provided a clear mark of success or failure in therapy. However, since streptomycin was of proven worth, it could not be withheld. Patients diagnosed at New York Hospital with whatever form of the disease were already receiving it, perhaps along with another antibiotic that was being evaluated. These drugs might have already altered the bacillus so as to make it more or less vulnerable to the test drug.

What was needed was a research population of individuals apt to develop miliary tuberculosis, who had yet to receive any chemotherapy. There was such a population in the US, but it was far from New York City and quite unknown to McDermott, despite his many years of concentrated work on TB. This population, about seventy-five thousand strong, was living on the 40,200-square-kilometre Navajo reservation in Arizona and New Mexico, where extreme poverty fostered high levels of disease and the rates of tuberculosis and infant mortality were the highest in the country.

In December 1951, a former colleague of McDermott's, Charles LeMaistre, then in the employ of the Epidemiologic Intelligence Service of the Communicable Disease Center, was sent to Tuba City, Arizona, to assist at a boarding school where three-quarters of the students had contracted infectious hepatitis. In the course of bringing this outbreak under control, LeMaistre learned that many tuberculous Navajo were going untreated. There was a tuberculosis hospital at Tuba City, but it was full. Patients with acute disease, including children, were being turned away, and simply went home to die without benefit of streptomycin because conditions allegedly did not allow the safe use of an injectable. LeMaistre brought this catastrophe to the attention of McDermott, who perceived in it the chance to conduct conclusive tests of isoniazid. He asked LeMaistre to approach the Bureau of Indian Affairs on his return to Arizona and request permission to bring the drug to the reservation. This was granted. McDermott was authorized to treat one child stricken with meningitis. He treated five, and two more with the miliary form of the disease, all successfully.

In February 1952, the results of the New York and Arizona trials were announced to the press. In March, the Navajo Tribal Council met with McDermott and asked him to begin a larger study at a one-hundred-bed hospital in Fort Defiance. From this overture grew an extensive and very ambitious program based on careful communication with elected Navajo leaders and with the traditional healers. McDermott and Kurt Deuschle, the director of the hospital, had the help of a woman named Annie Dodge Wauneka. Wauneka was the only female member of the council, and was appointed by them to help with a fundamental problem, namely the reluctance of patients to accept long stays in sanatoria. As of July 1953, of three hundred off-reserve patients sent to hospital in the preceding ten months, sixty-three had already left. Of the one hundred on-reserve patients at Fort Defiance, thirty-three were gone (Niethammer, 81). To prepare for her assignment Wauneka first spent three months studying at Fort Defiance hospital, a delay that caused some impatience in other council members. Having understood fully what she needed to convey, she visited the sanatoria and explained their illness to the patients, first informing them of the fact, news to many, that tuberculosis existed in all parts of the world and was not a uniquely Navajo disease. Patients were taken to the lab to view the "bugs that eat the body" (ibid., 91) on microscope slides, and shown x-ray films. Wauneka also collected tape-recorded messages from patients for their families, and vice versa, in order to ease the anxieties of all (ibid.). Subsequently she travelled the reserve persuading people to accept treatment. Early hospitalization was crucial. In 1939 and 1940, of three hundred forty-three admissions to Fort Defiance, two hundred thirty died. In time most participants in all positions came to see that not explanations of causes, but living proof of successful treatment – the return of people from the house of the dead – was the great persuader.

McDermott's team continued among the Navajo for ten years, trying the usefulness of isoniazid, PAS, pyrazinamide, streptovaricin and nicotinamide, and, after 1954, devising outpatient regimes. This last brought them again to the problems of patient compliance. In 1959 they were compounding isoniazid with riboflavin to enable an easy urine test to detect rejectionists. Another approach was the tamper-proof pill box in the form of a cylindrical device that patients rotated daily to extract medication (Jones).

After 1955, when responsibility for the health of Aboriginal persons was switched from the Department of the Interior to the Department of Health, Education and Welfare, McDermott organized an elaborate program that was headquartered in a new clinic built at Many Farms, Arizona. Physicians, anthropologists, nurses and linguists were brought together under the direction of the Cornell University schools of medicine and nursing. One of the initiatives carried through, corresponding to Knight's prescription, was that Navajo health workers were employed to remove the problem of poor interpretation. Eight of these health visitors were selected for training from among mature persons who had not been away at school or work for so long as to weaken their grasp of the language. Six of the eight had been hospitalized for tuberculosis. After four months of lessons and a year's apprenticeship, they worked in the field under a public health nurse, bridging the gap between the clinic and the scattered people.[28]

Of course the geographic similarities are slight. The Navajo Nation is large, and the weather sometimes severe, but distances in the Arctic are far greater, and conditions extreme. This is the most consequential difference. There were roads on the Navajo territory so it was possible to get to all corners of it, with difficulty. (When Arctic airways became well developed, health care practices in the North came to resemble those in use a decade earlier in Arizona.) Navajo religion was not displaced by Christianity but merely supplemented, and traditional healing practices were retained.[29] But also very important was the presence on the reservation of an elected tribal council – even if it was less independent of the Bureau of Indian Affairs than some would have preferred. To this body McDermott and company made their appeals and presented their arguments. What matters is not the scope of the Tribal Council's authority, nor how much knowledge of its deliberations was transmitted to remote camps, but the legitimacy of its voice among the people. After McDermott's initial success was reported, the council offered his team ten thousand dollars with which to continue their work on the reservation, on condition that the council receive a report as progress was made. Similarly in 1953, during a season of epidemic disease among that year's lambs, the council set up a price-support fund to buy and hold lambs that had been cured but could not be marketed immediately under the food safety regulations. Initiatives of this sort would have brought the council into good repute and won it a hearing on other matters, such as health. Whatever the limits on its autonomy from the American state, it was the council's communicative function that counted.

No such thing existed in the Eastern Arctic at that time. There were, to be sure, the old pan-Arctic organizations, in addition to the Department of Northern Affairs and National Resources. But the churches, the police and the traders all spoke *instead of* the Inuit, even when they attempted, as Bishop Marsh did, to speak *for* them. The coordination of all interests was supposed to occur, after 1953, in the Eskimo Affairs Committee, which met until 1962. Not until the tenth session, in 1958, were four Inuit invited to take part in a meeting of this body. (They were Abraham Okpik, George Koneak, Jean Ayaruark and Shingituck [also Shinuktuk or Sheenuktuk]. Also sitting in were Elijah Menarik and Mary Panigusiq Cousins [Tester and Kulchyski, 343].) Some time later the northern service officers organized community councils and co-ops, but Inuit political association really began in the high schools of Churchill and Yellowknife, whose graduates formed the Inuit Tapirisat, now the Inuit Tapiriit Kanatami (ITK).

In the 1950s, however, the Inuit had no political authority of their own to whom they could refer. But even so and even assuming the feasibility of northern hospitalization, and granted the will and the money, as Grygier puts it, nothing warrants that patients would have come in to those hospitals, or stayed once they had entered. Even among the Navajo, with the support of the Tribal Council and the Bureau of Indian Affairs, the tireless travelling and propagandizing of Wauneka and others, and the help from the health visitors, even with all that, persuasion and demonstration could not entirely overcome individualist and anti-authoritarian attitudes so far as to ensure that all of the contagious people accepted treatment. In 1958, the council debated for a day and a half before voting fifty-nine to six to request that the Public Health Service obtain from the secretary of the interior a regulation allowing the involuntary confinement of recalcitrant cases of contagious disease. In November 1961, the regulation came into force. How frequently it was used is not mentioned in the sources, but during the debate Wauneka claimed that there were eighty-five persons absent against medical advice in one small area alone (Niethammer, 117). And this was after six or seven years of coaxing and explaining. In the Arctic, the mode of patient transport, primarily ships operating on very tight schedules, effected quarantine without anyone having to explicitly invoke or enforce a law, although the possibility was often discussed.

There is another jurisdiction to consider before we leave this topic, and that is Alaska, where events largely repeated the Canadian pattern until 1955. A surge of postwar case-finding activity was followed by expanded treatment efforts, including the evacuation of patients by air to sanatoria in the Seattle area, once chemotherapy had begun to empty the beds. A hospital in Anchorage became the collection point from which people were routed southward, and by the spring of 1955 more than four hundred Aboriginal evacuees were in Seattle (Fortuine, 124). Efforts were concentrated in southeast and central Alaska, while there remained a greater problem in the North.

In 1953, the Alaskan Department of the Interior had commissioned a territorial survey from the University of Pittsburgh's School of Public Health. The resulting report, presented in 1954, asserted that the tuberculosis rates among the Aboriginal population in the north and west were extremely high: about 6.5 percent had active tuberculosis. The Pittsburgh experts then developed an ambulatory chemotherapy program (ACP) based on recent work showing the effectiveness of chemotherapy given on an outpatient basis in urban areas. The doctors decided to try this approach in the remoter parts of Alaska that were home to twenty-five thousand Yup'ik, Inupiaq and Athapaskans living in villages of about two hundred persons. Begun in January 1955, the ACP was at first limited to seventy-five villages containing about thirteen thousand persons (Fortuine, 137). INH and PAS were given to select groups in the hopes of arresting the progress of the disease in those who were infected, whether their TB was active or not, in order to reduce the need for eventual hospitalization.

Again, what allowed this program to go forward was the existence of institutional infrastructure that was lacking in most of the Canadian North at this time, including small hospitals, village schools and village councils. Chemo nurses were sent to the villages to meet with the council members and other local leaders, and request their assistance in recruiting a chemo aide, usually an Aboriginal, who functioned like the health visitors on the Navajo Reservation. The aide would talk to each patient every two weeks to ensure that the prescribed pills were being taken continuously and to assist the nurse in maintaining records. Close follow-up was necessary to ensure that resistant strains of the microbe were not being bred by intermittences in the treatments.

The Euro-Canadian approach to endemic TB among the Inuit varied with the therapeutic horizon. Until the advent of streptomycin, there were few TB evacuees. Serious cases taken into local hospitals were discharged to die at home. Strep permitted tuberculous Inuit to become candidates for evacuation, along with the seriously injured or gravely ill from other causes. However, until the emergence of the triple chemotherapy around 1953, people were taken south primarily to remove a source of infection from, and for the protection of, the immediate family and the local community. Concerns about the side effects of streptomycin, the possible need for surgery and the production of drug-resistant strains also entered into the balance. Removal for community protection was probably pointless, as the surveys of the early fifties found that almost everyone had been exposed. What mattered was not infection itself, but the conditions of life. Hunger, hardship and anxiety favoured the bacillus. After 1953, evacuation was probably preferred for reasons partly of efficiency (one thorough course of treatment was better than two or more less thorough passes) and partly from fears of the lurking resistant strain, as well as worries about the health-disfavouring conditions (deteriorating diet and housing) under which many Inuit were thought to be living. These considerations also influenced decisions about how long hospital stays should be. Here is the relevant page from the Indian and Northern Health Services Directorate Report of 1959, a compendium of extracts from regional reports:

> The duration of treatment for pulmonary disease is at least a year, but usually longer, and depends on
>
> a) Type of disease – Primary or re-infections, new or reactivation.
>
> b) Response to drugs – sensitivity of organisms.
>
> c) Complications – such as heart disease, emphysema, endocrine disorder, geriatric problems.
>
> d) Surgery – good or a poor risk.
>
> e) Co-operation – good or recalcitrant, personality disorders.
>
> f) In addition, poor environment conditions and the knowledge that out patients would not continue with the drugs at home influenced us to keep them longer to complete the standard regimen.[30]

A browse through the report provides an impression of keen and adaptable studentship on the part of those in charge. The doctors remained quite alert to new medical findings, and highly responsive to medical concerns, if not to social ones, which is a different story; that is to say, INH services were not administered in a rigid or mechanical way.

BCG use was still being modulated to fit changing circumstances. The central film library of the EAP was maintained in the regional office, and the x-ray films of previous years were supplied to the current patrol when it set out. The arrangement was pleasing to radiologists, who reported that comparison films made their work much easier and their fateful decisions (that is, to evacuate or take a chance on leaving doubtful cases behind) more reliable.

Failure cases emerged – that is, cases of disease resistant to strep or isoniazid – and something called cycloserine was tried, along with drugs to mitigate cycloserine's toxic effects on the central nervous system. Of seven "uncooperative patients" who took "irregular discharge" from hospital and were later readmitted, none showed any evidence of "deterioration of the tuberculous lesion" during their delinquency, and most of them had in fact improved. In addition, the reporter of this observation said, "I have felt for some time that statistics . . . have given quite an erroneous impression that the general tuberculosis program is being somewhat plagued by patients who leave hospital too early because they feel well when they are on drug therapy."[31]

The tone here is of a thoroughgoing and confident empiricism, a willingness to change one's mind when in receipt of new information and fit one's actions to new facts.

TWO: POWERS

1.

For twenty years (1950–1969) the flagship of Canadian aspiration in the Eastern Arctic was the Department of Transport vessel *C.D. Howe*. Every summer, the *Howe* carried the Eastern Arctic Patrol up the coast of Labrador, around the Ungava Peninsula, down along the east coast of Hudson Bay, across to Churchill and finally north to Baffin Island and higher latitudes before returning to Montreal.

The November 2, 1947, memorandum to cabinet proposing a new vessel for the government's Eastern Arctic Service resumed the case for the expenditure in seven points. Two had to do with medical services and research, one with sovereignty and one with defence. The dimensions and facilities of the desired ship were set out, and the operating costs estimated. Assuming annual steaming of about 32,200 kilometres, these would be on the order of $150,000 to $170,000. (In 1945 the Hudson's Bay Company supply vessel *Nascopie* did about half that mileage for $55,000.) The new ship would be owned by the Department of Transport, would operate north of Hudson Bay and would be required to service a growing number of installations in the high latitudes if necessary. Three years later, in September 1949, the *C.D. Howe* was launched by Cabinet Minister Howe's daughter-in-law, and in June 1950 was commissioned by the Coast Guard and set off for her first northern tour.

The *Howe* replaced the *Nascopie*, which, crewed by Newfoundlanders under Captain T. F. Smellie, had supplied the company's eastern posts for the previous thirty years. In the words of a southern medical emissary, the Toronto surgeon Dennis Jordan, the voyages were through "uncharted waters . . . when radio was in its infancy, radar unknown, airplane travel hardly begun; when the successful annual voyage of this ship was the one yearly contact of the Eastern Arctic with the outside world, and when the failure of the ship to get through meant privation and hardship to both Eskimos and white men" (quoted in Wild, viii).

The end for the *Nascopie* came on the afternoon of July 21, 1947, when the ship struck a reef at Cape Dorset, came off at high tide, then went hard aground again about three in the morning and stuck fast for some months before vanishing into deeper water (Wild, 192).

Nascopie's replacement for Eastern Arctic Patrol purposes was a brand-new ice-strengthened vessel designed by German and Milne of Montreal, and built by Davie Shipbuilding at Lauzon near Quebec City. The *Howe*, an instrument of new policies, was owned and operated not by the HBC, to whom the Canadian government and the medical and scientific communities had been beholden until then, but by the Department of Transport (and then, after 1962, the Canadian Coast Guard). The ship entered government service in 1950 and continued as the medical patrol vessel until 1969.

The *Howe*'s primary mission however was resupply. (In winter she serviced navigational aids in the Gulf of St. Lawrence.) In 1960, thirty-three vessels moved ninety thousand tons of cargo, including large quantities of fuel oil, to northern outposts.[32] Air resupply was also a huge undertaking. Operation Boxtop, carried out in 1963 by Hercules aircraft shuttling between Thule and Alert, involved two planes flying around the clock to carry more than fifteen hundred tons of cargo, two-thirds of which was fuel, across 1,300 kilometres. To reduce loading time, the fuel was transported in neoprene "blubber bags," five to a plane (Royal Canadian Air Force).

Steel-hulled and ice-strengthened, the *Howe* was an advance in reducing the distance that both allowed and required the autonomy of northern dwellers. The chief obstacle to sea travel in the Arctic was ice and, in some circumstances, almost every ship would be defeated. Fred Lee, who was aboard the *Howe* in 1957, recalls the vessel becoming stuck in ice at Lake Harbour (southeast Baffin Island) with a good wind packing ice in upon her. Escape was impossible until the wind went around and moved the ice away again. Neither the *Howe* nor the Hudson's Bay Company ship was able to reach Igloolik (northeast of the Melville Peninsula) that year (Tippett, 25). It was usual to send the *d'Iberville*, a true icebreaker, to the higher latitudes at the same time as the *Howe*, to assist if needed. The better idea was to go over the ice by plane, or under it, and by 1960 there were regular submarine voyages by American naval vessels (Thorén, 4). On March 17, 1959, the US nuclear-powered submarine *Skate* surfaced at the North Pole in order to conduct a memorial service for the Arctic expert Sir Hubert Wilkins. "In compliance with one of his last wishes, his ashes were then scattered in the driving snow" (Gagné, Northern News, 121).

Air ventures in the vicinity of the North Pole were not uncommon even before the war. In August 1937, a four-engine monoplane left Moscow heading for Mexico over the top. Five hundred kilometres beyond the North Pole, the pilots radioed a report of engine trouble. Nothing more was heard from them. Sir Hubert Wilkins organized a flying search out of Coppermine that continued for thirty days, and then after a break for refitting, resumed with a new plane and went on by moonlight until March. In total the search covered some 54,700 square kilometres of territory north of the Arctic Circle. Two years later the Hudson's Bay Company bought a twin-engine Beechcraft and that summer, Sir Patrick Ashley Cooper, the governor of the company, and two of his top managers were flown from Edmonton to Winnipeg, making surprise visits to twenty-eight posts on the way. Although *routine* does not quite apply, there was certainly great confidence in air travel in the north from about 1940 on. By 1950 an RCAF Dakota (a military configuration of the Douglas DC-3 airliner) could fly a medevac mission from Edmonton to Eureka on the north shore of Ellesmere Island and down to Churchill in three days, covering 5,800 kilometres in that time (Ellis, 338–39).

Planes carried medical services into the Western Arctic all through the fifties and sixties, and came into ever greater use in the Eastern Arctic as well, until the medical patrol was switched entirely to aircraft in 1969 or 1970. By then ninety percent of the people, previously semi-nomadic, were concentrated in permanent settlements, and nursing stations existed at four points on Baffin, as well as at Igloolik. Small aircraft using skis or floats were more dependable because they were more flexible with regard to weather.

As for the *Howe*, she was sold to Cominco and sent by a subsidiary, Vestragon Mines, to Greenland. There she served as an accommodation ship for the Black Angel Mine on Affarlikassaa Fjord. In 1974, while en route to ship breakers in Spain, she was purchased by another mining outfit in a deal brokered by Marine Salvage of Port Colborne, ON, and registered to Windward Shipping, but nothing seems to have come of this venture, and after a delay the ship was almost certainly broken at Castellón de la Plana, Spain, in 1974 or 1975.[33]

The ship, and its equipment, was an important means by which Canadian administrators consolidated and exercised their authority over the hinterland that had become a focus in the global balance of military preparedness. The mobilization of non-military science, technology and medicine, and its delivery into the North by way of the *Howe* and other supply and research ships *is* the politics of this period.

2.

The *Howe*'s helicopter was the first to be carried on a non-military vessel, and for purposes of the mass TB survey proved indispensable. The innovation required tuning however. The original helicopter, a Sikorsky, was lost on the *Howe*'s maiden voyage into the north. The replacement was a Bell 47, the bubble-nosed craft familiar as the American medevac vehicle of the Korean War. An early example, the Bell-47D1 from 1945, hangs in a stairwell at the Museum of Modern Art in New York. This machine was in production for thirty years, and more than five thousand were sold. Canadian air service companies were eager early adopters. Lundberg-Ryan Explorations, an Ontario prospecting outfit, ordered two machines after test surveys in 1946, and sent pilots to Buffalo to train with Bell. The next year, a third machine went into action as a crop-duster in Southern Ontario, and four more went west to do the same. By the mid-sixties, there were two hundred twenty-six Bell helicopters at work in Canada – more than half of all the machines registered as civil aircraft (Petite).

The Bell design is owing to Arthur Young, a mathematician and theosophist who, dissatisfied with his first attempt at a unified cosmology, decided to turn his mind to something narrower. Casting about for something to constrain his thought within the bounds of a specific physical problem, he selected the helicopter as his focus because it was a stalled yet clearly desirable and attainable advance, and in 1928 set off on a twenty-year voyage through the difficulties. With him went engineer Bartram Kelley, who continued in the aircraft industry as a Bell vice-president when Young returned to his philosophical interests in 1947. Kelley described the situation when he and Young began as follows:

> A great variety of machines was designed and actually built by people who were not content with the growing development of the airplane, and were striving toward the goal of hovering flight. The fortunate inventor would gather sufficient financial backing to construct a full-sized machine. He would concentrate his energy on the mechanical problems connected with rotor drives and structure, and also on obtaining sufficient lift, assuming that if the craft once took to the air, his troubles would be over. However, they were just beginning. In most cases the machine would refuse to stand still in the air, and would start to tip and move, oscillating back and forth in an ever-increasing swinging motion, often in spite of the best efforts of the pilot. There is one historical record of the instability becoming so violent that a machine finally landed exactly upside down. (685–90)

Young and Kelley worked with small-scale remote-controlled models in order to sort through errors rapidly. Eventually they achieved steady flight by means of a stability bar mounted to the mast below the rotor by a see-saw pivot and linked to the rotor hub in a way that allowed the bar to vary the inclination of the rotor with that of the mast, but with a delay.

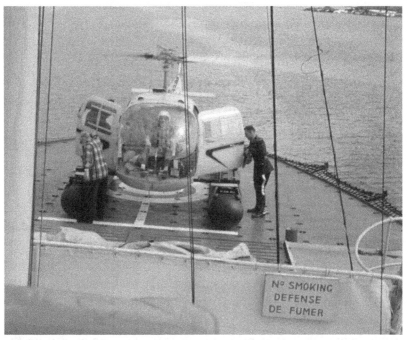

Bell helicopter on the deck of the *C.D. Howe*. Courtesy of the Archives of HHS & FHS, Johanna Rabinowitz Fonds.

Once the practicability of rotating wing flight was proven, the helicopter proliferated rapidly and many designs emerged. The Canadian Navy icebreaker *Labrador*, for instance, launched in 1951, carried either two single rotor Bell HTL-4s or a Piasecki HUP twin rotor. But the Bell remained the darling of civilian users, the staple default all-purpose vehicle.

Commenting in 1955 on the usefulness of the *Howe*'s Bell, John S. Willis was enthusiastic:

The benefits of the helicopter were vividly brought to my attention on reaching Sugluk. Father Verspeek, who came aboard and had a chat with me in my cabin before the anchor had been down ten minutes, informed me that there was a camp four miles away containing a number of sick, in particular a girl of about twenty who was coughing blood and very weak indeed. Dr. Schaefer was sent off immediately by helicopter and returned an hour later to say that there were two camps close to one another, with several sick. The helicopter was sent again, this time with Miss Anne [*sic*] Webster, the nurse, who brought the patient back safely. By boat this trip would have taken far more time and jarred the patient a good deal, besides involving much more strain on the personnel. I was most impressed.[34]

The core of the medical enterprise carried into the North by the *Howe* was its x-ray capacity. This enabled the rapid diagnosis and speedy evacuation on which the whole eradication program depended; and on the reduction of TB and other infectious diseases depended all other plans for rearranging the lives of northerners.

By the mid-forties, the evolution of x-ray techniques had suggested the following logic to anti-TB combatants. Since the rest cure was the only demonstrated treatment at that time, and since the more active the case, the more contagious it was, it followed that early detection would help with both considerations: the earlier the burden on the patient was lightened, the better the chance of recovery, and the sooner he or she was removed from close contact with others, the less the chance of transmitting the bacillus. The lung, with its high contrast between air and tissue, is a natural for x-ray examination. Hence, as x-ray devices became safer and more stable, the images more readable, trained personnel more numerous and exposure times shorter, the hope of scanning a sizeable portion of the entire population became realistic. The final analysis then was a) the comparison of the cost of case finding by radiography versus that by other means, and that of treatment after the disease had sufficiently expressed itself to cause the sufferer to themselves seek help; and b) the acuity of x-ray technique compared to other clinical methods of detecting the disease.[35] The results of the analysis in this country were provided in the *Canadian Journal of Public Health* in 1955 in the form of a table of "Case-finding Activities in Canada, 1944 to 1953." In 1944 mass surveys screened about four hundred thousand persons. Thereafter the trend was always up, until, by 1953, two and a quarter million people were seen, with another six hundred thousand passing through clinics (Wherrett, "Recent Developments in Canada's Tuberculosis Services").

Even before 1944 there was a great deal of activity. The troops were x-rayed from 1939 on, and war workers as well. Another few years, and the procedure was so cheap – fifteen to twenty cents a person for miniature films – that it became ubiquitous. Many companies had an x-ray done of all new hires. Hospitals made it part of admission procedure.

Saskatchewan, ever the leader among Canadian regions, had begun to x-ray entire communities in 1941. Ontario and Manitoba followed. By 1950 Saskatchewan had done two

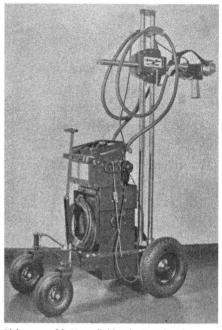

Picker portable X-ray field unit. © Colonel A. A. de Lorimier, Army School of Roentgenology, Memphis, Tennessee, in Lawrence Reynolds, "The History of the Use of the Roentgen Ray in Warfare," *American Journal of Roentgenology* 54, no. 6 (December 1945): 665, figure 20.

sweeps and was about to start a third. However, some were still being left out. Fixed x-ray sets were fine in larger towns and cities. Mobile equipment was taken into rural areas as far as there were roads to run it on. But beyond the end of the road were the scattered Aboriginal communities of the boreal and Arctic regions. To reach them with this equipment, especially in the Eastern Arctic and along Labrador, it had to be truly portable, and this was the contribution, in the first instance, of the Picker X-Ray Corporation of Cleveland, Ohio.

This company was founded by James Picker, a Russian immigrant to the US, who trained as a pharmacist in New York City and shifted to the x-ray business after becoming an agent for the sale of Kodak plates to users of the new apparatus. In 1929, Picker, a daring man, purchased an important equipment manufacturer named Waite & Bartlett and also the assets of the Engeln Electric Company, a prominent maker and designer of x-ray devices, and started a plant in Cleveland. Picker developed a sales and service force, and began to manufacture equipment, as well as continuing to deal in supplies and accessories. Things went well. Picker gave his line a stylish, moderne look by using chrome, colour and streamlining on the first product, a vertical fluoroscope offered in 1931. By 1937, the company was responding to a design call from the Belgian army to develop a piece of equipment, presumably portable (Palermo).

Two years later Picker's son, Harvey (later president of the company and eventually a health care activist on the international stage), wrote to the Surgeon General of the United States offering to design a field unit that would no doubt be needed should the US enter the war. The result was the US Army X-ray Field Unit, a wheeled machine a little larger than a man, which collapsed into three chests (five, counting fluoroscopic attachments and the transformer) and could be assembled in five minutes. Design criteria included a maximum weight per chest of two hundred pounds, which could be carried by two men. The set was extremely versatile. Film processing equipment along modular lines was also provided, and Picker engineers produced a sixty-cycle gas-fuelled generator whose output corresponded to the requirements peculiar to x-ray generation (de Lorimier and Dauer). Picker engineered and prototyped this product, bid on its mass production, won the contract and subsequently trained another manufacturer to build it in order to provide the customer with a second source. Thirteen thousand units were put out, earning about four million dollars that James Picker returned to the Department of the Treasury, with the remark that "I did not want to make a profit on men dying" (Palermo, 110).

Immediately after the war, the Picker machines began to move north. Already in 1945 George MacCarthy and Campbell Laidlaw, reporting on the southern portion of the Eastern Arctic Patrol (Montreal to Churchill) conducted from the *Nascopie*, complained of the lack of the apparatus:

In accordance with request, we attempted, as best we could, to ascertain how prevalent tuberculosis is among the Eskimos. However, as most of the patients brought to us were suffering from a variety of other conditions, our study of this particular disease was extremely limited . . . the handicaps of our being unable to make a wider clinical survey in the time at our disposal of being without X-ray equipment were unfortunate. It seems most important that all the natives should be examined carefully both by X-ray and otherwise in order to find out how many are harbouring tubercular foci . . . by using an aeroplane and a large motor boat, a physician and a technician with portable equipment might be able to go over the whole field during the summer months.[36]

Out west, Don Harkness, the technician in charge of the radiology department at Camsell and of surveys conducted from that base, recalled for the Charles Camsell Hospital history committee that the department possessed, in 1946, one 220 milliamp fixed unit and one portable. In the late summer of 1947 he was able to acquire a second portable, likely a Picker, and an American army ambulance. The first mass survey undertaken with this equipment was at Hobbema (now Maskwacis, AB) in September 1947. At the same time William Anthony Paddon, at North West River in Labrador, was struggling with few resources to deal with "a bottomless pool of tuberculosis patients" (Paddon, 117) and no beds for them, there or in St. Anthony. Paddon's coasting vessel, the *Maraval*, had been refurbished, and he now purchased a Picker Portable X-ray, and operated this machine, which proved "reliable and indestructible" (ibid., 119) for the next twelve years. During the first summer, he took one thousand one hundred chest shots, which "gave us our first accurate impression of the scope of the problem we faced . . . From then on we X-rayed everyone over three years of age once a year, comparing the film with the previous ones each season to detect even the smallest change" (ibid., 119–20).

Back in Edmonton, Harkness obtained one of the new photo-fluoroscope machines:

In the winter of 1947 funds were made available to purchase a new X-ray unit manufactured by Picker X-ray, a 70 mm machine designed to do mass surveys. The principle on which the unit was designed was to have the patient fluoroscoped, then a camera would take a photograph of the fluoroscopic image. The camera contained a 70 mm roll of X-ray film and would allow a technician to take approximately four hundred and fifty X-rays per roll, thus eliminating the need to set up a darkroom to change the film after individual X-rays. This allowed us to X-ray up to one thousand persons in one day. (Charles Camsell History Committee, 133)

A photograph in the City of Edmonton Archives from March 1948 shows three technicians and their truck, with a large gas or diesel generator in tow. Shortly they were off to the Blackfoot reserve where one thousand four hundred people were surveyed in two days (ibid., 134). After this Harkness organized the hiring of summer help (pre-med students) and ran four surveys a year.

Meanwhile the EAP doctors got their wish and during the 1946 voyage of the *Nascopie* a survey of "all Eskimos available" was done. The equipment was a Picker portable "complete with generator."[37] All but two hundred of the films made were processed on board, another first. Reading of the shots however had to wait until the medical party got back to Ottawa, where a team of three experienced chest specialists viewed them. Reckoning with an estimated population of six thousand, the doctors thought they had sampled pockets representing about three thousand seven hundred. Of these, thirteen hundred forty-seven or thirty-six percent were x-rayed. All age groups were sampled, except for children under five.

Noting that "this was the largest number of Eskimo films to have ever been obtained," the doctors felt able to make a few judgements. First, that "the Eskimo is pretty thoroughly tuberculized" in all areas. But also, that "there seems to be ample evidence that the Eskimo shows a marked resistance to tuberculosis. The widespread evidence of previous infection showing gross calcification with no evidence of activity seems to bear this out." This implies that active cases would respond readily to treatment, that is, to rest and adequate diet. In conclusion, "it would seem that the Eskimo presents no special problem in the way of tuberculosis control inherent in their particular race. They have evidently been tubercularized for many years and have survived as a race in spite of a high morbidity and mortality rate and with no attempt made to treat or segregate open cases ... The problem then is the environment and the mode of life of the Eskimo, plus the present insurmountable transportation dedicatees."[38]

In the Western Arctic it was 1950 before surveying among the Inuit began. Attention went first to the Yukon, where in one operation seventeen thousand were examined. The first attempt at a mass survey involved a doctor and two technicians who were flown into Cambridge Bay by the RCAF. The team then jumped around from this base using a Norseman bush plane with skis. Of the nine hundred fifty-two x-rayed, including twenty-five non-Inuit, seventy were brought out for hospitalization.

When the *Howe* took over from the *Nascopie*, she carried a portable unit along with the fixed set in the hospital section of the ship (supplied by Picker, probably from their branch in Montreal). The *d'Iberville* also had an x-ray machine, which was mentioned by Simpson in his 1952 EAP report. The next major shift in EAP x-ray procedure occurred in 1955 when John Willis became Indian Health Services Regional Superintendent, Eastern Region. The limits of what could be done from the *Howe* were to be surpassed by initiating a saturation survey with immediate evacuation – that is, sequestration of positive cases, who would then be conveyed to the nearest point from which they could be taken south by air. To that end, four additional medical parties would be dispatched to cover ground that the *Howe* could not. Presumably all four carried x-ray sets of some sort. Films were to be read wet, on the spot. And so it was done, for a decade, with extra medical parties eventually yielding to year-round nursing stations, and air transport steadily gaining over ship travel. Concern about stray radiation and overexposure of the medical people and their patients, as well as electrical hazards, recurred throughout the working life of the *Howe*, and the struggle with the equipment and procedures seems to have never ended. On completing the 1950 tour, the radiologist insisted that the x-ray apparatus be given its own dedicated converter, to avoid fluctuation of the current when other demands were on the line. When the four hundred sixty-three films collected in that year were read at Parc Savard hospital, they were deemed not as good as previous films. Technicians were advised that women should not be allowed to let their braids hang down their back, believing that the braids "have doubled the difficulties of giving an accurate X-ray reading in about 50 to 55% of the films. They produce shadows very similar to those of an exudative process and in the upper parts of the lungs in about the same regions usually invaded by an incipiens [sic] tuberculous focus."[39]

Assuming an accurate interpretation could be made, many films were not meaningfully identified because the technician's version of this or that person's name was impressionistic and therefore useless unless a disc number was also provided. (These identity disks featured an intaglio of a crown, the legend *Eskimo Identification Canada* and a two-part code. One part indicated the district where the disc was issued, the other a number unique to each individual.) Keeping the shots in order from year to year, and making sure they got onto the *Howe* each spring to allow comparison was still a stumbling block in 1957. And perhaps the radiologists had become more demanding. Joseph Lee, on board that year from Quebec City to Resolute, complained that the x-ray machine was one of low output, necessitating long exposure times. In a letter, he wrote, "This time varies according to the thickness of the chest, which in an Eskimo is usually considerable. Also occasional bone X-rays are attempted. With the inability to adequately explain procedures to the patient because of language difficulties, various errors occur which are exaggerated because of the long exposure time."[40]

Lee recommended a switch to a faster film, which would halve exposure time; faster intensifying screens, which would halve it again; and a new, faster developer as well.[41] Whether Lee was heeded or not, the following year's team x-rayed an amazing 2,269 persons and conducted complete physicals on 1,571 of them.[42] Most importantly, the films of previous surveys, properly labelled, should always be shipped with the medical party.[43] However, in 1959 the INHS Annual Review of Medical Services claimed that this problem was solved by the Central

Film Library in the regional offices. "On the Eastern Arctic Patrol, where films are taken, developed and read, the films of previous years are made available from this library for comparison. Radiologists are pleased with this arrangement and report that comparison films make their work much easier and their fateful decisions (i.e. to evacuate or take a chance on leaving doubtful cases) more reliable."[44] The *Howe*'s fixed set was replaced at least once, probably in 1959, and perhaps again in the mid-sixties during the mass migration to solid-state equipment.

The helicopter and the x-ray apparatus revolutionized medical care (hence politics) in the Eastern Arctic. The helicopter allowed authority to go where it otherwise could not, to take in doctors and nurses, and to bring out the sick and the injured. X-ray machines allowed the delineation of the true scope of the TB problem. They also gave the doctors greater confidence in marking for assimilation into the medical system persons who otherwise would not present themselves for examination, since they showed no symptoms, or, if examined, would not be readily diagnosed; nor, if diagnosed, accept treatment. However, these appliances had to be taken north from their southern places of manufacture, and for that other developments were required: ships and planes able to move cargo reliably across great distances through extremes of weather. In the Western Arctic, x-ray machines went by road, by river-going boat and ultimately by plane. In the East, transport through the fifties was mainly by ship.

The principal fact of life in Canadian waters is ice. The further north one goes, the more of it there is, and the thicker it becomes. The master of a vessel that is proceeding through ice-bound waters attempts first of all to make way through open channels between quantities of ice. When these leads peter out, the ship's progress depends upon the strength and shape of its hull, and the power of its propulsion system. Hopefully the bow rides up on the ice that breaks under the ship's weight. (To this end, the front end of the *Howe* was loaded with concrete.) The shape of the bow then determines which of the secondary problems will arise: large slabs of ice slamming the propellers or travelling into the ship's wake to obstruct any vessels that the icebreaker may be leading, or smaller chunks building up ahead of the ship, which eventually halt its progress.

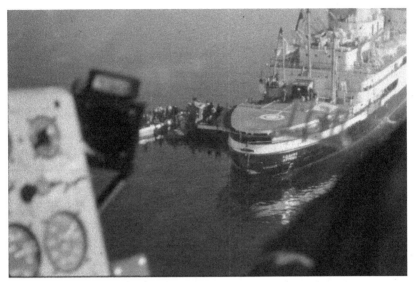

The *C.D. Howe* from the helicopter it carried. Courtesy of the Archives of HHS & FHS, Johanna Rabinowitz Fonds.

The *Howe* was ice-strengthened, built more to follow leads rather than to break ice – as befit a vessel meant for resupply and the provision of services, and which had a fairly southerly itinerary. By comparison *Howe*'s sister ship, the *d'Iberville*, an icebreaker, was half again as large but had almost three times the propulsive power.

Finally, new navigational aids, in particular radar, eased the anxieties of Arctic mariners. Astronomical navigation had always been vague, due to the faults of compasses and the limits imposed by weather that obscured celestial bodies and/or the horizon required to calculate a position. Radar helped to locate islands and large icebergs, as well as the headlands of landfall in conditions of low visibility.

3.

During the first few years of the modernized EAP it was often rough going, and things remained chancy through the fifties. The impression received on going through the records is one of doctors and administrators who had bitten off a good deal more than they could chew, even when the weather conditions and other circumstances were not set against them. Often they were.

As a concrete expression of political ambitions the *Howe* was useful. As a medical vessel, she was misconceived. For most of the ship's working life the resupply missions took precedence over other functions, forced the pace of medical work and truncated it when people were not immediately at hand on the ship's arrival. Early complaints were that the *Nascopie* had stopped for two full days at each port of call, while the *Howe* paused for perhaps one day, and then half the work had to be done after dark. Without the helicopter, much less would have been accomplished. The *Howe* raced from wharf-less port to wharf-less port, getting in where she could as weather permitted and off again likewise, and the medical teams examined whatever portion of the populace the

local notables (nurse, cleric, policeman) had managed to assemble or the helicopter pilot could find and ferry into x-ray range. Quite soon the ship was supplemented by other vessels and increasingly by aircraft. Already in 1953, of thirty-nine patients scheduled for repatriation after release from hospital fourteen were going on the *Howe*, four on the *d'Iberville* and twenty-one by air.[45]

There were three principal authorities on the *Howe*: the

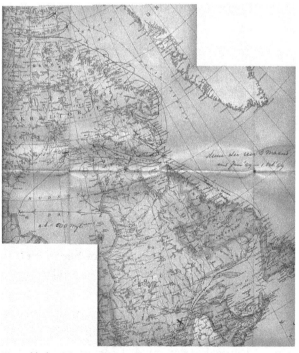

Map with the *C.D. Howe's* 1958 Eastern Arctic Patrol itinerary marked. Courtesy of Johanna Rabinowitz scrapbook, private collection.

captain, the chief medical officer and the officer in charge of the Eastern Arctic Patrol overall – the government's representative, the man in charge of administrative concerns. This individual actually functioned as an observer and rapporteur for purposes of providing reliable information to planners. All three reported on their work, and all three sets of documents have made their way largely intact into the national archives. The captain filed a daily log of arrivals and departures, miles steamed, fuel consumed and so on. The medical and administrative officers filed preliminary reports as they went along, and also composed a final report. These were day-to-day accounts of difficulties met and tasks accomplished, apparently worked up from journals, and contain many interesting details about conditions in the communities visited and often expressions of strong personal opinion on what should be done about what was seen. Many are highly readable and at least one, R. A. J. Phillips' hundred-page report on the Montreal to Resolute portion of the 1955 patrol, is of literary merit as well as great historical interest.

The civil service entry procedures had yet to be modernized, so the crew at first were recruited anew every year, and had little training or experience (Grygier, 94). During the first leg of the *C.D. Howe*'s very first trip, the helicopter was lost. On August 5, 1950, the Sikorsky aircraft dropped into the Koksoak River (which empties into Ungava Bay) immediately after takeoff. Sam Ford, a seventy-year-old interpreter from St. John's, vanished with the machine, and his body was not recovered with the wreckage. The pilot, Charles Parkin, and civil servant Gerald Johnston, who was acting as an assistant to Alex Stevenson, the officer in charge of the patrol, were rescued (Bailey, 36). The following year the replacement machine was a Bell 47. The ship reached Quebec at the end of September, with the Catholic mission ship *Regina Polaris* (disabled at Sugluk Inlet) in tow (Stevenson, 19).

In 1952 Paul Fournier took over as captain. The ship hit an iceberg off Labrador and had to return to Quebec City for repairs. There, the shipyard workers were on strike, so Fournier had to proceed to Montreal. It was August 2 before the patrol was resumed from Quebec City, making the ship a month late and forcing the cancellation of twenty-five days of a planned one-hundred-day (19,300-kilometre) trip and the elimination of five of the scheduled twenty-one ports of call. Even so, one hundred twenty-nine active cases of TB were found. The 1953 trip, again under Johnston and Stevenson, seems to have gone more smoothly, but Bent Sivertz, chief of the Arctic Division of Northern Affairs, went along in 1954 and was very unhappy with what he observed.

Sivertz was a navy man, an instructor in navigation and the commanding officer of the navy's officer training school during the war. On the *Howe* he noted that fire and lifeboat drills were rare or sloppy. Fire instructions were in English only, while the crew were francophone and many passengers spoke Inuktitut. The ship was dirty. Officers and crew drank too much. Freight was misdirected. Navigation procedures were inadequate and antiquated, owing to a lack of qualified personnel, and so on (Grygier, 95). Moreover, a review panel convened in the fall of that year concluded that while the *Howe* had visited an average of eighteen ports of call in each year, at which a total of 3,511 persons were "on the average reasonably available for examination," only an average eight hundred ninety-two of these, a mere twenty-five percent, had in fact been examined. The trouble was that the people weren't reasonably available. In fact, people were usually living some kilometres off from the Euro-Canadian outposts (store, church, RCMP post), in part because sternly paternal whites discouraged Inuit from tarrying too near the company and its stores, lest they become spoiled for the rigours of the semi-nomadic hunting life. Although people tended to come in and congregate at shiptime, it seems this was not always the case. Assembling all of the locals before the ship came in to allow the greatest number of examinations during the usually very limited time, perhaps a day or two only, did not often go smoothly. In addition to the *Howe*'s ports of call, numerous camps in the Eastern Arctic were home to another 2,459 persons (the figures derive presumably from the 1951 census), none of whom it was possible to examine at the medical facilities on the ship. (When there was a place to do so, the medical team would set up on shore, with the generator-powered portable x-ray equipment.) Even when identified, not all active TB cases had been adequately addressed. Sivertz was told by a missionary at Cape Dorset that of twelve Inuit scheduled for hospitalization the year before, none had been evacuated and five had died. The remaining seven were to be moved on to Iqaluit in September.[46]

What to do? It was not possible to increase the time spent in each port. And anyway, "if a substantial increase is to be achieved in the number of persons to come in, as much field organization would be required to bring them in as to take the medical party to them." There was to be no stepping back from the goal. To this end, in April, the eventual medical officer on the 1955 trip, John Willis, tabled a plan of saturation survey: "The topography of the Arctic divides Eskimos into groups which cannot easily come into contact with each other. Disease in one group is therefore not readily transmitted to the next. By doing a separate saturation survey on each group, removing all cases suffering from infectious disease, tuberculosis being the main problem, it should be possible to effect in a few years a noticeable improvement in the health of the people."[47]

Willis was anxious to establish strict routines for the medical parties to allow reliable comparisons between the findings from one year to the next. The chief innovation, however, had to do with the diagnostic procedure:

> One of the difficulties of previous surveys has been that X-rays were taken on a given group, the films taken south, and the positive cases not identified for some weeks or even months after the X-rays had been taken. By this time transportation difficulties of the winter season had arisen and it became almost impossible to get out these cases. This summer it is proposed that the X-rays be taken and developed on the spot, that the films be read while still wet, and that positive cases be brought out immediately. To do this, transportation sufficient or [sic] up to 5% of those examined would have to be provided together with rations and other stores. The idea would be to convey these positive cases along with the medical party to the nearest point from which they could be flown south.[48]

This is the inception of the classical picture of the *Howe*'s activities, and the 1955 patrol marks the turning point in the battle against the disease.

Sivertz, Willis and Phillips were newcomers in Arctic circles. They were possessed of great energy and eager to take things in hand, to identify and resolve problems. These three, along with Walter Rudnicki (welfare services) and perhaps Donald Snowden (housing), drastically reformed the management of Arctic affairs. A Toronto graduate, Willis had served a two-year stint with the British Colonial Service in Hong Kong before becoming interested in the North. In October 1955 he became general superintendent of Northern Health and continued in that position into the sixties ("Among Those Present"). Phillips was brought into northern administration after spending the immediate postwar years in the Soviet Union, and then a year as an instructor at the Royal Military College of Canada in Kingston, ON. These two had their own opportunity to assess first-hand the work done from the *Howe* the year after Sivertz. Together with Rudnicki, who was engaged from 1956 in developing social welfare efforts, these men reorganized medical and other services and obtained, as the phrase is, many efficiencies. In 1959 for the first time more Inuit were returned home than were evacuated.[49] More tellingly, of the three hundred twenty patients brought out of the Eastern Arctic, two hundred fifty did so not in consequence of the EAP survey, but as a result of continuing surveillance by field staff.

Willis divided the territory, the Eastern Region, as he called it, into five areas, each to be served by its own survey party, consisting of a medical officer in charge, a male nurse or medical student, an x-ray technician, an interpreter and possibly a dentist. The first group was to ship on the *Howe*, the second was to visit the south coast of Baffin, the third would go to Quebec and Ungava, the fourth would do the lower part of Hudson Bay and the fifth would cover the coast of Labrador. It followed that the *Howe* would have to be supplemented with the Department of Transport ice patrol vessels.

Other shortcomings were also being addressed. The *Howe* design called for accommodation for fifty, including four women. In 1955 the four were Ann Webster, of Coppermine, the adopted daughter of Archdeacon Webster; Paulette Anerodluk, also from Coppermine; and Joan MacArthur and Lois Long of Ottawa. Webster had a nursing degree from Victoria and had been out of the North for many years, most recently with her parents in England. Unfortunately she was diagnosed with appendicitis during the first leg of the trip, and was ordered ashore at Churchill for surgery in southern Canada (Hankins, 60). Anerodluk had trained as a nursing assistant in Fort Smith, NT, and had herself been hospitalized for TB of the lungs and hip. She had lost her parents and some siblings to the disease (ibid., 60). MacArthur was to function as a secretary, and Long performed as a laboratory and x-ray technician. MacArthur's position, later termed *registrar*, was essential for the detailed record keeping that Willis instituted on this trip.

Before joining the ship, Webster and Anerodluk visited Mountain Sanatorium (probably at the behest of Sivertz) and gathered messages from patients to be delivered to their families along the *Howe*'s route. In another step toward improving the hitherto poor communication between the medical patrol and the population the doctors brought along a film made at the Mountain San. Willis recorded it being shown to an audience of eighty at Port Harrison (now Inukjuak). Technical problems persisted. The transformer that converted the ship's 220-volt direct current to 120 alternating to supply the x-ray equipment failed, and a new one had to be ordered in to Churchill.

> The equipment in the Hospital Unit is in a poor state of repair. There was no power in the operating and X-ray rooms for 24 hours after sailing and none in the dentist's office for 48 hours. The water supply in the dental room was off for three days after sailing. The autoclave and the instrument sterilizer leak badly and the pressure gauge on the former is out of order. The X-ray tank overflow pipe leaked at the lower joint and had to be mended with rubber dam borrowed from the dental kit. The cassette holder has been repaired twice and the viewing box three times. Our trouble over the power supply has already been communicated to you by telegram. I

have been so thankful that I brought a tool kit along – I have used every item in it, including the soldering iron, to keep the equipment functioning.[50]

Elsewhere in this confidential report written during the usual layover at Churchill, Willis spoke very well of the four women, especially praising Anerodluk. He also set down a good account of the procedures with which the medical team received its clients.

Probably the worst trip was had by Dr. H. B. Sabean and his team in 1957. There was overcrowding, with up to ninety persons in the Inuit quarters and sick bay, in space made for fifty. Sabean felt it was wrong to leave seventy-six repatriates hanging on at Churchill waiting for transportation when the *Howe* was on its way to their destinations, so he took them aboard. A large group got off at Coral Harbour as expected. However, those who were to land at Lake Harbour were prevented by an outbreak of measles on board. The ship continued to Resolute and all Inuit were put off to a quarantine camp. "This location I recall only as somewhat of a nightmare," Sabean reported.[51] The disease was contained however, and the patrol resumed, now down to one nurse, no nursing assistants, no interpreters and one other doctor – supplemented by volunteers recruited from among the passengers. Alex Spalding and Alex Stevenson, an old HBC hand and now a government man, pitched in.

In charge overall during the first leg (Montreal to Resolute) of the 1955 patrol was R. A. J. Phillips, who had already spent March and April touring the Central Arctic by air.[52] Phillips was an important figure at Northern Affairs from 1954 on, when he came in from the Privy Council (in fact, he even named the department) (Robertson, 113). His background was in the Department of External Affairs, following wartime service in the Canadian Intelligence Corps. He spent most of his career near the top of the bureaucracy, usually in the near vicinity of Gordon Robertson. In April 1957 Phillips became chief of the Arctic division. Along with his other duties he was first editor of *North/Nord*, the division's bimonthly review, in which capacity he styled himself The Rajah. Barry Gunn, a Scot who went to teach at Cape Dorset, met the higher-ups in Ottawa in 1956, and observed that "the whole

Department, and that certainly included the Education Directorate, was ruled over by R.A.J. Phillips. Although Bent Sivertz was at that time Director of Northern Administration Branch, it seemed to me that it really was the RAJAH who was running things" (quoted in Macpherson, 129).

North/Nord was the organ of a policy clique that articulated the administrators' aspirations for their domain. These changed over the course of a decade or so from integration to assimilation, a change discussed by Alan Rudolph Marcus and more fully by, among others, Tester and Kulchyski, and Damas. As a writer Phillips was suave and engaging. When addressing a closed audience of his peers in a confidential report, he sometimes indulged a wicked wit. At Eskimo Point (now Arviat, NU) during a 1955 flying inspection he found Mr. X "luxuriating in the exhilarating cynicism which follows a letter of resignation,"[53] while "Bearded Father Ducharme rambled gently down the paths of his experience as he sat in pyjamas by his glowing coal fire."[54]

A few months later Phillips was on the *Howe* as officer in charge, going as far as Resolute, and described the trip in a hundred pages. In this travelogue-cum-diplomatic dispatch, produced for a restricted readership, he was at his liveliest.

> Five minutes after we began our two mile boat journey, the "HOWE" was completely obscured by fog and in ten minutes it was obvious to even the dullest of us that we were completely lost. We could see neither the ship nor the shore and the visibility was probably no greater than fifty yards. So we continued zigzagging this way and that across Hudson's Bay on a trip bearing more and more resemblance to the last voyage of the man who gave it his name. Any historical parallels were rudely interrupted by a thundering crash as we hit a reef. The waves reached lasciviously for our gunwhales and the motor sounded like the interior of our sick bay – a deep silence punctuated by heartrending coughs. We eventually got off and the skipper of our craft announced to me that we could head for shore. This was a sensible course of

action, if only we knew where the shore was. We headed off in some direction with two men hanging over the prow with a pike pole. So we sped off into the fog. I make no claim to any knowledge of navigation but no one will convince me that we were not at that moment headed straight into the open sea . . . By the sheerest co-incidence in our westward crossing we happened to pass below the stern of the "HOWE," close enough for someone to see a light. And so we were able to continue the patrol, and the local parson was deprived of the biggest service Harrison had ever known.[55]

As an essayist and pamphleteer the Rajah was more restrained, though still very readable. He published in venues as diverse as *Queen's Quarterly, External Affairs, Canadian Architect* and *Weekend* magazine; contributed to *The Idea of North*, the first documentary of Glenn Gould's Solitude trilogy; and for some years wrote a column for the *Ottawa Citizen.*[56]

A dedicated colonial administrator, he could also be obtuse when official. Here is his treatment of events so calamitous for the Inuit victims that they have prompted entire volumes of investigation: "On the basis of local advice, but without any opportunity for objective resource surveys, the people were taken from Ennadai Lake northwards, to live around Padlei. It was no use. The suffering continued. Means of supervision over the dispersed people were almost totally lacking. Disaster struck more quickly than news could travel" (Phillips, *Canada's North*, 174). This economical paragraph is about the Ahiarmiut deaths at Henik Lake in the winter of 1957/58, and the starvation deaths at Garry Lake in the same winter. These were episodes of bungled intervention and were almost certainly chastening for Phillips as for the rest of the divisional brass, though no one seems to have turned up any remarks to that effect on paper. In any case, not chastening enough to deter them from proposing another relocation, which eventuated in the village of Whale Cove, high on the western shore of Hudson Bay. It is not clear if Phillips failed to see how badly his division had handled things, or if he saw but refused to publicly make an admission that could have been costly to the department.

Instead the bureaucrats were able to turn the public's distress over their errors to their favour, as has been documented by Alan Rudolph Marcus, by combining secretly with Farley Mowat to assist the folksy writer in the development of his crusader persona.[57] The Minister of Northern Affairs and National Resources, Alvin Hamilton, Sivertz and others mouthed a few acts of contrition and extracted an increase in funding.

Willis, who was Phillips' counterpart at Health and Welfare, held a diploma in Public Health from the University of Toronto's School of Hygiene. The school was the child of Connaught Medical Research Laboratories and remained closely related to it (Bator and Rhodes, xi). In 1947 the diploma program consisted of 1,040 hours of instruction with courses in bacteriology, immunology and serology, parasitology, virus infections, biometrics, epidemiology, communicable diseases, physiological hygiene, industrial hygiene, public health services, public health education, sanitation, chemistry in relation to hygiene and public health nutrition (ibid., 111).

Willis would have gone through something similar in 1950. It is safe to say that he was sensitized to the role of infectious agents in human illness when he went north in 1955. There, he wrote,

> I saw baking powder, Johnson's baby powder, dirty spoons and forks, pieces of meat and fat, dirty clothes, a basin of flour, a half-moon type of Eskimo knife, empty tin cans, and a clock, all together on a crude table, in the "kitchen area" of one tent. Yet in others, one would find all the items neatly arranged in groups, according to their functions. It seemed [to] be a common habit to place the meat in a pile in a corner behind a row of stones, on the opposite side of the tent from the sleeping platform . . . In summer at least the toilet seems to be the great outdoors, where I saw men urinating without shame in the open before their people. The women appear more modest. That there seem to be no camp rules about the disposal of excreta is borne out by the fact that I observed dried fecal material strewn about at random all over the camp site but usually not within ten feet of a tent. Although I have

been told that the dogs consumed the excreta I have not seen one doing this yet. Possibly it is done in winter when food is scarce. The camp sites I visited were littered with odd bones and even partial skeletons of animals, as if the meat had been hacked off without dismembering the carcass, the bones being left to the dogs to pick clean . . . We saw implements loaned from tent to tent, food borrowed – bannock for my evening snack at Koartak came from another tent, brought in with willingness and reverence by an urchin with hands as black as my boots. Chewing gum is passed from mouth to mouth and a cigarette passed around the family circle when tobacco is in short supply. The mothers chew food for the infants. Tuberculosis is thus shared by all.[58]

There is more to be said about the last-mentioned practice, however, which usually was begun with babies around four months old, and as medical knowledge grew, crude opinions like these gave way to a more sophisticated appreciation of Inuit methods.

Otto Schaefer, an internist trained in Germany, emigrated in 1951 and did a tour on the *Howe* in 1955 and again in 1957. By 1959 he had come to understand, for example, the importance of the Inuit infant-feeding practices that had dismayed Willis in 1955.

The early mouth-to-mouth feeding of small amounts of pre-masticated meat and fish, boiled as well as raw, may be another effective factor preventing scurvy and rickets and providing all important nutritional elements including iron. This is started in breast-fed babies usually at four to five months, to be followed later, when the baby has enough teeth, with small morsels of fish and meat. The bulk of nutrition, however, is derived from the mother's milk until the next baby takes, after about three years, its place on the breast. I have seen several well-developed Eskimos, adults and children, who were pointed out to me as having been exclusively brought up with mouth-to-mouth feeding from the very first weeks of life, after losing their mother post partum or being given away as a twin (an Eskimo woman can keep only one of twin babies, for there is only room for one in her parka). (Schaefer, 386)

By 1964 Schaefer had worked for many years in the Arctic and at the Charles Camsell, and was head of a new Northern Medical Research Unit headquartered in Edmonton. In that capacity he reorganized the way examinations were conducted and recorded in order to prepare a program of clinical research. It was proposed "to use observations made during the Easter time survey in Western (Central) Arctic and during the Eastern Arctic patrol as a general orientation to gain clinical impressions comparative to observations during the years 1953 to 1957, and to serve as a basis for planning future field studies with particular regard to the suitability of certain population groups and local facilities for detailed investigation of specific medical, physiological and biochemical problems."[59]

Although Schaefer was careful to note that the medical services were much better in 1964 than in 1955, he also found a good deal wanting, even with the basics. While acknowledging the limits of what could be done with the *Howe*'s cramped space and poor equipment, he emphasized that blood and urine checks, done for the first time on this tour, could and should be performed every year. He was perplexed to find that the treatment of ear infections was haphazard, with both antibiotic and non-antibiotic drops used and no attention given to fighting the underlying disorder. The drug supply was inadequate, and he thought that in particular antibiotics for ears and pediatric iron tablets should always be on hand. He was also worried that pregnant women might be receiving exposure to stray x-rays, either when having their own chest film taken or when holding their children. Since it was not possible to know at a glance whether any woman was pregnant or not, he recommended that all should be fitted with a protective apron.[60]

In short, ten years after the patrol's reorganization following Sivertz's criticisms, the quality of care being provided was still, in the opinion of someone who was certainly qualified to judge, rather mediocre.

4.

What was it like then, to be among the members of the medical party on this ship in the mid-1950s, during the heyday of case finding, evacuation and repatriation? The medical people, in company with their colleagues from the bureaucracies, were awed by the beauty of the landscape, often dismayed by the conditions of life they saw when they went ashore, and sometimes overwhelmed by the work, which came in intense bursts. They were frustrated by the deficiencies of the *Howe*, which was chronically under- or ill-equipped from a medical perspective, and whose schedule made them rush what should not be rushed or omit entire communities from the survey. They had strange encounters and close scrapes. John Willis, helicoptered to a camp somewhere on Diana Bay near the end of day, was stranded overnight when fog closed in. It was early on his first trip. After giving a shot of penicillin to a child with a draining ear, and receiving indications that there was no other sickness in the camp, Willis "reasoned that if there were no more sick to treat, perhaps I should spend my time trying to learn how the healthy kept that way in this environment. As they were very friendly, I started over the rocks to the far end of the camp, hoping to work my way from tent to tent as a friendly visitor. It was about nine o'clock by this time and the scene was so quiet and strange that I had the sensation of having been suddenly planted in a moon world inhabited by friendly gnomes" (22).

R. A. J. Phillips ornamented his report of a visit to Wakeham Bay with this picturesque description: "Shortly before 2:00 a.m. we left the ship still 10 miles off shore. The helicopter is not licensed for night flying and this was as close to night as we ever used it during the trip. Flying in was one of the most remarkable air experiences of the journey. The helicopter itself was dark, there being no lights even on the instrument panel. The sky was dark blue, the ship 500 feet below ablaze in the luminescent sea. The northeastern horizon was being split by bands of cold red light and ahead the plastic hills rose up a thousand feet."[61]

Murray Ault, writing of his feelings half a century after his 1959 tour as a cabin steward, spoke in terms of "the mystery and grandeur of the Arctic."

We had been at sea for ten weeks and had re-crossed the Arctic Circle. We were headed south. I had not been to the stern of the ship. This had been off limits and perhaps for good reason! It was a cold, clear night . . . I decided to take a surreptitious tour . . . As I stepped onto the deck, there, stretched out behind the ship, was the shimmering white wake as it disappeared into the total blackness of the night . . . It was a mesmerizing sight as the moonlight caused the wake to sparkle brightly . . . I moved closer to the stern and the galaxy above was in full view. I could easily find the North Star, the Milky Way and the Dippers . . . off in the distance I could see the loom of the land. There was a glistening on the cold steel deck plates where I stood. I could hear the faint rumble of the engines below and feel the vibration of the propellers . . . The sound of the water sliding past the ship and the splashing sound of the wake close to the stern as we made our way broke the mystical silence of the north. As I listened to these sounds, they added a special silence to the scene.[62]

On his return Ault had the photographs he had taken mounted as oversize slides. Fifty years later, these are fading to magenta, futile attempts to contain vastness, but still convey some sense of the emotion felt by the voyager in the presence of the sublime immensities that the camera failed to capture.

Up until 1945, the *Nascopie* had carried a doctor only. After that, it carried a doctor, a dentist, one eye surgeon and an x-ray technician (Grygier, 88). In the earliest days of the revamped Eastern Arctic Patrol, the medical party consisted of two doctors, a dentist, a nurse, an x-ray technician, a dispenser and a sick-bay attendant. This group managed to see about eight hundred of the likely two thousand Inuit at that time residing on Baffin Island (Brown, 491). (There is uncertainty about the numbers. Another report on the 1950 survey of Baffin gives the number seen as five hundred ninety-eight rather than eight hundred.) Parallel surveys were being made at James Bay and in the Western Arctic. Thirty-five hundred persons of all races were x-rayed around James Bay. Among eight hundred fifty Inuit, fifty-seven were found to have active tuberculosis ("Tuberculosis Survey," 141). However, the Western foray of 1950 was not very comprehensive, and large numbers of people were not surveyed until 1953.

By 1958 there were two or three doctors, a dentist, two nurses, two nursing assistants (both Inuk), a radiologist, one or two assisting technicians, a dogsbody who assisted the assistants and a social worker – a position added in 1957 to insure that provision was made for family responsibilities to be reallocated before the patient left.

In 1957 the junior officer was Fred Lee, the nineteen-year-old son of one of the doctors on board. Lee had a yen to go somewhere far. He had applied for a spot on a trip to the Antarctic, as well as on the *Howe*. (He later joined the navy.) Since the doctor in charge of the EAP that year was Sabean, who had spent the spring at the San working with Lee's father, his chances of acceptance were good. According to Murray Ault, all of the cabin stewards and junior technical assistants owed their placement to influence. However, the job was no sinecure. Lee's principal task was to develop x-rays. This he did in a little darkroom adjacent to the x-ray room, handing the films back to be read wet. This was not ideal, and required experience in the readers, Lee's father and his colleague Dr. Peart. (Each of these men served for half the trip. Churchill was the usual switching point; later, Resolute.) But speed was essential since an immediate decision had to be made as to whether the patient would be returning to shore that day or staying aboard for evacuation. In the evenings Lee Senior would review the now-dry films, in case anything had been missed, but by then it would be too late to do much about it. When skiagraphing Inuit lungs – and little but chest x-rays were done – it was necessary to "hit them hard," that is, to increase the dose in order to obtain a good shot with those very deep-chested people. But not too hard, since overexposure would eliminate soft tissue detail, making the film unreadable. Rarely, the younger Lee would find on processing that the shot was poor, and the technicians would retake it.

Those being examined were quite patient, once they were on board, although some tried to evade their would-be benefactors altogether. The entire ship's company was also x-rayed, and in all about eight thousand shots were taken over a four-month period.

As Lee recalls, the Inuit smelt strongly of fish oil. Murray Ault experienced similar olfactory distress, "Eskimos [are] really funny . . . unfortunately they stink some."[63] They were especially odoriferous of foot, when their boots came off, but impressed the medical team with the perfection of their skin, which was very smooth and without blemish. Otto Schaefer remarked in a 1959 overview of his Arctic medical practice that impetigo due to scratch infections was common, but that psoriasis and eczema were never seen among the Inuit. As for fish oil, his praise was unstinting: "sea mammals and fish . . . are rich in *unsaturated* fatty acids . . . and are often shunned by whites for their repugnant smell. We seem to have lost the healthy instincts and natural senses of primitive peoples, who often crave rancid oxygenated (unsaturated) fats. Baffin Island Eskimos have a special treat in summer, namely, Arctic char (a species of salmon with an extraordinarily high fat content) sewn raw into sealskins and exposed to the sun for two to three days. By fermentation and oxidation, they thus instinctively enrich the unsaturation of the fatty acids" (Schaefer, 387).

When not in the darkroom, Lee had other duties. He was charged with ensuring that meals moved from the galley to the Inuit quarters. He enlisted a few adolescents to help him fetch the food in trays and pails over the many stairs and ladders. At Resolute, a major supply drop, almost all the Inuit patients were put off the ship for a week and their accommodations given over to stevedores flown in to unload three ships. There were Inuit women in the sick bay and Lee remembers being told to watch over them and ensure they were not troubled by the stevedores – an assignment that kept him sleepless for a week.

By 1962, the medical party had grown to twenty-five, when the social work contingent was counted. The doctors had been joined by an ophthalmologist and an ear, nose and throat specialist. There were five or six nurses, two dental technicians, and various translators and assistants (Grygier, 100). By 1964 attention was turning to the so-called epidemiological transition, and Schaefer was aboard collecting information toward eventual research into cardiovascular status and pulmonary functions in older men with regard to diet, smoking habits, obesity and other factors.

In 1958, the year that Johanna van der Woerd (who later married Paul Rabinowitz) participated, the complement was two or three doctors, one of whom was Lee Senior back for a second half-tour; two nurses, Van der Woerd and Iris Crandell; two nursing assistants, Mary Panigusiq and Maggie Hatuk; a social worker, Betty Marwood; and the radiology personnel.

Marwood was taking over from Ruth Banffy, who had been the inaugural social worker. Banffy had ended seven years of improvisation, during which it was left to the nursing assistants and whatever other Inuktitut speakers might be on hand to communicate their diagnosis to prospective evacuees and help sort out some part of their affairs at the very instant of their sudden departure. Of these assistants in 1958 Maggie Hatuk was a weak Inuktitut speaker, probably having lost her language in hospital as a young child.[64] Mary Panigusiq's adventures had begun around 1944, when, at age five, she was aboard the RCMP ship *St. Roch* during part of its celebrated voyage through the Northwest Passage from Halifax to Vancouver. Panigusiq boarded at Pond Inlet along with her uncle Joe Panipakoocho and five other members of the family. Joe was taken on as insurance – should the vessel become icebound and the crew have to overwinter, an Inuk guide and hunter would be very useful indeed. Mary hated the trip, was anxious about living in a tent on deck and loathed the food. The Inuit disembarked at Herschel Island, YT, in September, and were picked up again the following August by the eastbound *St. Roch*. It took another year to reach home (John Beswarick Thompson, 78). According to an article in a 1959 issue of *Time* magazine, at twenty Mary was editor of *Inuktitut* magazine and a major contributor of copy and drawings, having done four years of schooling in Hamilton. There are photographs of her modelling a fur coat (for Eaton's), conferring with Iris Crandell and Betty Marwood on the *Howe*, posing with her parents and siblings at Grise Fiord and making her listeners laugh at a diplomatic reception in Ghana, where she spent six weeks as a goodwill emissary. In 1966 she was living at Grise Fiord and married to a schoolteacher named Roger Cousins, while apparently working as a radio journalist. Later she was at Buffalo Narrows, SK, for a time, and shortly before her death in 2007 was living with two daughters in Ottawa. Obviously an intriguing bicultural figure whose personal path paralleled that of Eastern Arctic history in the second half of the century.

Also aboard for some portion of the voyage were Terry Ryan (who appears in Van der Woerd photos), Alex Spalding and James Houston, who appear in a collage of Panigusiq's pictures published in *Inuktitut* magazine. All three were members of that anomalous band of men and women infatuated with the North, who were neither missionary nor policeman nor organization man, but who made themselves very useful to Inuit and Ottawa men alike during the Great Transition.[65] Ryan, a young artist and Ontario College of Art graduate, came aboard at Clyde River, where he had just spent two years at a radiosonde weather station as officer-in-charge (Tippett). He was at the beginning of a lifelong association with the people of Baffin Island, where he assisted in founding the West Baffin Eskimo Co-operative and was seminal to a branch of the Inuit culture industry.

Spalding was an HBC man whose account of his northern apprenticeship, *Aivilik Adventure: A Reminiscence of Two Years Spent with the Inuit of the Old Culture*, contains many carefully, indeed lovingly observed details – often with Inuktitut vocabulary attached – of day-to-day life in and around Repulse Bay in 1946 and 1947.[66]

Spalding was quite another kind of mind than Phillips. Both more scholarly and more poetic, he could allow himself the following:

> I had another *big* dream about the white whales, close cousins of the dolphin . . . I dreamt this one many years after I had left the North and while I was working extremely hard at university to pass my exams. This was a very vivid and very meaningful experience to me, and for days after I felt in the

most wonderful health and disposition and I was extremely creative and fruitful. I had looked into the eye of God so it seemed, the eye of his benign aspect . . . We were going through deep earth caverns and, reaching water, I now saw myself astraddle on the back of a white whale which turned to let me know or warn me that we were in for a sharp climb. While I was hanging on to its back, it made a sudden and tremendous leap, and the cliff wall seemed to heave and shake. I felt myself falling back – a desperate feeling! . . . But the whale came and held me up, and smiled at me with the most marvellous love and goodwill – a beatific vision! – and I then felt totally confident and serene as we broke through the surface of the water into the sunlight! (Spalding, *Aivilik Adventure*, 222)

Van der Woerd was fairly new to the country, having come from Holland with a sister in 1954, not particularly intending to stay. By the time she went aboard the *Howe* at Montreal in June 1958, she had already been a year and a half at Moose Factory General Hospital, a posting she sought after the first Aboriginal patients from the James Bay region began appearing at Mountain San. For her, the *Howe* trip was continuously eventful with moments of high emotion and a great deal of work, strain and anxiety. There were occasional shore leaves, with hikes and evening singalongs, and some adventure as well – a walrus hunt (a whale hunt she declined) ending in success, the butchering of the beast and the obligatory morsel of raw meat, carefully selected so as not to make her sick, and having a sort of nutty flavour. A different sort of decorum was maintained at dinner on the boat, with the men donning suits and ties and the Mounties their scarlet tunics, as can be seen in Van der Woerd's photographs. The ritual of the Arctic Circle crossing was observed, with certificates duly signed by the captain issued to first-timers, the celebrants dressed up in whatever costumes could be found, and Neptune enthroned and attended by two mermaids. One of these was Panigusiq, who appears in photographs of the proceedings with a frizzy blonde wig atop her dark pageboy cut. A certain amount of drinking and flirting went on, although Van der Woerd reported that serious attempts at philandering on the part of married medical personnel were thwarted to the best of her knowledge (personal interview).

The good times were interspersed with some very difficult ones. Dr. Lee began to look poorly. Confined to his cabin with intestinal bleeding, he was brought x-rays to read while lying on his bunk. At night Van der Woerd slept below, providing morphine as it was requested. Simple blood tests confirmed that he was quite ill, but his return south was delayed by troubles with the communications owing to a burst of radio-jamming solar activity. R. Hayward, a Southern Ontario zone superintendent for Health and Welfare who wrote the medical report for 1958, described the circumstances:

> There was a microscope provided but no key to open the case. There were no slides, coverslips nor substage lamp. There were no stains for bacteriology. Doctor Van den Berg tried hard to get blood for Doctor Lee but had no typing sera. The carpenter cut some microscope slides out of the glass from a picture frame donated by the First Officer. Several people said they had Group "O" blood which was supposed to be Doctor Lee's type. After laborious spinning of their bloods in the hand centrifuge it was found that cross-agglutination [indicating no match] occurred in every case.[67]

Van der Woerd flew out with him to Churchill – not in the helicopter but in another plane. From there he was taken back to Hamilton, where he died of cancer shortly after. At Sugluk a seaman with a severe head injury was transferred to the *Howe* and thence by air with Van der Woerd at his stretcher to Churchill, on the far side of Hudson Bay, which was reached at midnight. As no other nurse was available, an already exhausted Van der Woerd had to assist in surgery – ultimately unsuccessful in saving the patient's life. The return to the *Howe* was made on a small plane equipped with a pail for a toilet. The distress of patients who were diagnosed as actively tuberculous and obliged to stay aboard when others went off was troubling, as was the parting from children whom she had known or cared for at the San, and who were now returning to places that they did not themselves feel was home. To her parents Van der Woerd wrote, "I dropped one of my patients home to her tent. She had been 3-½ yr in the San. She was now 9 years & it was difficult to say goodbye. She wanted to come back with me. Spoke very little Eskimo and did not recognize her family."[68]

Most of all, there was a great deal of work – continuing, in Van der Woerd's case, all the way back to Hamilton, to which she escorted Inuit without assistance from Montreal on. Willis wrote during his 1955 trip,

> There is a tendency for some of them to forget that they are not on a cruise to Hawaii, feeling that they should be given shore leave at every port. On the other hand, I have proved to myself that after four hours hard work examining Eskimos crowded into the very narrow passageway and hospital rooms, the efficiency of the team goes down and the quality of the work suffers. Generally therefore we work four hours on and two hours off . . . Documenting the work properly, putting up requests for repairs, meeting with the team to iron out snags, repairing equipment, and attempting to be nice to the 'whites' on shore, takes up all my time and energy . . . My attempt to read Churchill's memoirs, which I brought along for the leisure hours that seemed so obvious from a look at the ship's itinerary, have failed miserably.[69]

The procedure, as organized by Willis in 1955, continued much the same each year thereafter: after those to be examined were assembled on deck, one family at a time was admitted to the hospital unit passage, where "an interpreter sits just inside the door of this cabin . . . and takes down on a Family Record form the name, disc number, year of birth, infancy history and diseases history, usually from the mother."[70]

These discs had a two-part code. One part indicated the district where the disc was issued, the other a number unique to each individual. The discs are usually accounted an affront to Inuit dignity by Inuit and Euro-Canadian commentators. Eventually the disc numbers were dropped, but instead of simply replacing them with social insurance numbers and leaving Inuit naming practices to revert to tradition, Ottawa at the end of the sixties undertook Project Surname (Alia).

Valerie Alia has gone into the matter thoroughly. The problem was the difficulty that both Euro-Canadians and Inuit had with each other's naming systems. Inuit solved it by simply renaming Euro-Canadians with whom they had to deal. For example, Spalding became Titirarti, the writer/clerk; Gimpel was Bearded Seal; Leo Manning was Ijiki, small eyes (Tester, McNicoll and Irniq, 128). James Houston was Saumik, Leftie.

Euro-Canadian renaming of Inuit was more various. There were first of all the spelling troubles. Mary Panigusiq was also Panegoosho, Panikapushoot and Panegusiq, depending on the orthography of the day, not to mention Mary Cousins (her married name), as she was identified in her Inuit Tapiriit Kanatami obituary of 2007. Christianizers urged, and Inuit converts accepted, baptismal names, with similar spelling vagaries. Thus Mary could yield Imellie (Alia, 27). Bob takes an *ie* ending to make the word more Inuktitut sounding, and loses the non-Inuit *b* to become Poppie. In the mid-1930s the police began a system of fingerprinting, not carried through. The fibreboard identity tag, suggested by military usage, went into service around 1941. Unfortunately, and quite predictably, the assumptions underlying the disc system could not hold. People moved about. Discs were lost or forgotten at home. An adult might remember his or her number, but children might not. Sivertz told Alia that "there was a problem identifying people who did not have discs or had lost them. It was difficult to assign [people who had been sent out to hospital] to a family or a community, without the discs. There were a lot of children who were lost because nobody bothered to send their discs with them" (44).

Nor is this the only mention of this particular problem. Bishop Marsh, writing to Gordon Robertson (the then deputy minister of the Department of Northern Affairs and National Resources) in 1954, asserted that P. E. Moore had "publicly stated" that there were fifteen

Inuit children who were unidentified, could not speak Inuktitut and could not return home because no one knew whence they had come.[71]

Next, continuing with Willis's account, "As each name and disc number is recorded, the interpreter places opposite them, on the Family Record form, a serial number. At the same time this serial number is written with a blue ball-point pen on the back of the left hand of the Eskimo concerned. This number serves to identify him quickly throughout the medical examination."[72]

This family record form, a sample of which was bound into Willis's draft plan, was lengthy, and was to be completed "on each family encountered, and on each individual encountered who lives apart from his family, e.g. orphans, men out hunting away from their families." In an ecstasy of punctilio, Willis indicated that "it will be seen that, when the right hand portion of the form is folded at the vertical line separating 'Skin' and 'Eyes,' bringing the right hand edge level with the double line adjacent to the heading 'Sex,' the folded form is 8" wide and 5" high, and may be filed as an ordinary filing card."[73]

Presumably this document remained on the boat, but what happened when the boat returned south in September, perhaps bearing one or another member of the family while the others remained in the North? Van der Woerd remembers that x-rays went to Ottawa over the winter, and then were placed on the *Howe* again the following spring. Did the family record accompany them? The business is obscure, and becomes more so when considered alongside the complaints about people becoming lost in the system – that

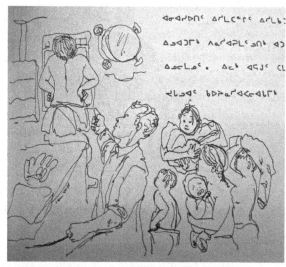

X-ray examination on the *C.D. Howe.* © Mary Panigusiq Cousins, *Inuktitut* magazine, 1959. Courtesy of Inuit Tapiriit Kanatami.

is, being off somewhere in southern Canada without the family being told where, precisely, or in what state of health.

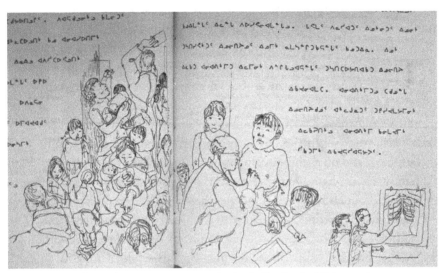

Medical examination on the *C.D. Howe.* © Mary Panigusiq Cousins, *Inuktitut* magazine, 1959. Courtesy of Inuit Tapiriit Kanatami.

At step four, a fourteen-by-seventeen-inch x-ray photo was taken.[74] Next, "the family passes, one by one, in serial order, to the Operating Room, where they undress and are examined stripped following the routine: Mouth, Eyes, Vision, Ears, Hearing, Skin, Nutrition, Chest, Heart, Abdomen, Neurological, Limbs, Genitals. An assessment of emotional stability has been attempted where information was available, and cleanliness of person and co-operation were recorded."[75] This was a lot to do, requiring a good deal of concentrated attention. No wonder Willis's team found it tiring.

Step six was a dental examination, and seven was a blood sampling. Eight was vaccination with a diphtheria-pertussis-tetanus mixture prepared by Connaught Laboratories. Connaught was as much a part of the industrial base as Davie or Vickers, and had been since the Great War, when it produced two hundred fifty thousand doses of tetanus antitoxin for the troops, and smallpox and tetanus vaccines as well. By 1928 it was in the business of preparing sixteen biologicals, including insulin (Bator and Rhodes, 37). A round-the-clock operation with one hundred forty workers turned out five thousand 400cc bottles of blood serum every week in 1941. Blood donations climbed until by war's end two and a half million had been collected and processed (ibid., 73). In 1945 a million doses of typhus vaccine were produced every month.

Diphtheria infections occur usually on the skin or in the respiratory tract; if the latter, it appears as whitish exudate on the tonsils, caused by cell-killing toxin. In a day or two, this substance develops into a grey, adherent membrane. Attempts at removal cause bleeding. The membrane may spread, and the toxin travels in the blood to do damage in the heart, nerves or kidneys. In 1923, Gaston Roman, working at the Pasteur Institute, obtained a diphtheria toxoid – the toxin treated with formalin and heat to render it non-toxic but still able to stimulate the immune system to fabricate antibodies. Connaught brought this toxoid into large-scale production, and this was the *D* component of the DPT administered on the *Howe*.[76] The *P* and the *T* are pertussis (whooping cough) whole cell killed vaccine and a tetanus toxoid, respectively. *Bordetella pertussis* first of all attaches to the cilia that sprout from the lining of the windpipe and the bronchial tubes, and serve to transport foreign material out of the airways into the beyond. "The paroxysmal cough results from inability to expel tenacious mucus; the whoop is created by vigorous inspiration through the glottis at the end of the paroxysm . . . During paroxysms, cyanosis may occur" (Mortimer, 536). This goes on for four weeks or so, with or without all manner of complications – pneumonia, encephalopathy and so on. About half of affected infants under three months die. Five-year-olds almost always make it through. What the EAP nurses were giving against pertussis was a whole cell vaccine. The whole cell preparation contains unknown quantities of irrelevancies and things reactive – that is, they cause the human frame to flinch chemically. They stimulate inflammation, which is non-specific, and the complementary immune response, so that the recipient of the vaccine experiences redness and swelling at the injection site, some pain from the swelling and some fever.

Tetanus (*Clostridium tetani*) is a spore-producing creature that resides in the soil. When the spores are introduced to soft tissues under low-oxygen conditions, they germinate; by and by, when the resulting bacillus dies and disintegrates, the host receives a dose of tetano-spasmin, a toxin that travels to the central nervous system and interferes with its normal reflexive apparatus, effectively damaging the off switches. Sufferers from generalized tetanus present with spasms of the jaw muscle, or with raised eye-brows and clenched eyelids, or with sudden contractions of all muscle groups, and/or the heart can be thrown off beat or sped up. *C. tetani* is dangerous most of all to newborns, entering at the umbilical cord stump. At present, neonatal tetanus accounts for eighty to ninety percent of *C. tetani's* victims. The toxoid is made by purifying cell culture medium and neutralizing the toxin with heaping helpings of formaldehyde, most of which is then removed. Bringing the diphtheria toxoid, the pertussis vaccine and the tetanus toxoid together in one preparation reduces the number of needles that the recipient has to tolerate.

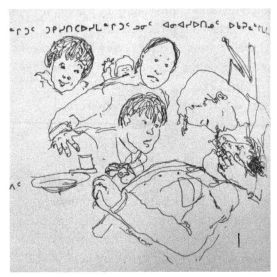

Dental examination on the *C.D. Howe*. © Mary Panigusiq Cousins, *Inuktitut* magazine, 1959. Courtesy of Inuit Tapiriit Kanatami.

Writing an overview a couple of years later, Willis indicated that the battle was far from won. By 1957, he said, it was not TB – which killed fourteen Inuit in that year – but acute respiratory infections that were the most serious health problem, accounting for the majority of the two hundred thirty-eight Inuit deaths overall. Of these deaths, one hundred seven were infants.[77] Almost a quarter of Inuit born alive died during their first year and at least half of these deaths were due to respiratory disease. That would be diphtheria, pertussis and influenza, with pneumonia likely intervening. For adults, especially adult males, lined up on the *Howe*, however, it is hard to see what was gained by vaccination, except perhaps some tetanus protection. Likely it was simply easier to give everybody the same injection, and the procedure was probably thought helpful in another regard: the Inuit were being initiated into patienthood, trained to accept the ministrations of doctors and nurses.

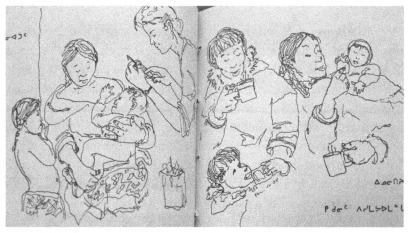

Vaccination on the *C.D. Howe*. © Mary Panigusiq Cousins, *Inuktitut* magazine, 1959. Courtesy of Inuit Tapiriit Kanatami.

In addition to DPT, Willis had on hand Bacille Calmette-Guérin (BCG), the TB vaccine, and the polio vaccine. The BCG was reserved mostly for the very young, because the x-ray survey was showing that almost everyone else had signs of TB in their lungs.[78] The polio vaccine was in short supply – he had three hundred courses after Port Harrison – and was held aside for Resolute and Frobisher Bay (now Iqaluit), presumably places with nursing stations. The next year, all were given the polio vaccine, and were inoculated with smallpox as well – unless they had the scars of a previous encounter with the bug, or were to receive BCG. Smallpox immunization was complicated and required close attention to perform correctly:

After cleansing the skin over the region of the left deltoid with ether and allowing to dry, expel the drop of vaccine contained in the capillary . . . Using the sterile needle supplied, make 20 to 30 skin punctures <u>through</u> the drop without drawing blood. Then, holding the needle parallel to the skin, move it in a circular fashion, exerting gentle pressure meanwhile . . . Do not dress the site of vaccination. If possible, the patient should be warned that a systemic reaction can be expected later. He should also be warned to leave the scab alone.[79]

As persons processed through the line, about fifty in a session, "it was found helpful for each officer to record his work on the left hand of the individual, the dentist recording a 'D' on the palm . . . the nurse a 'B' for blood and an 'X' for toxoid," et cetera. The following year this was modified to X for x-ray, P for physical examination, I for immunization and D for dentist, on the right. By the time D was done, the X-ray film would have been read, and the patient was then marked with an arrow under the XPID, signifying negative for active tuberculosis and free to go. When tuberculosis was found, the XPID legend was underscored in red, and TB added beneath. "NO ESKIMO TO LEAVE SHIP WITHOUT CHECK OF RIGHT HAND," screamed Willis's Administrative Guide for 1956.[80] To round out the proceedings, a film was shown and a box lunch distributed. The Inuit reportedly liked them both, particularly the film made at the San of patients from Baffin.

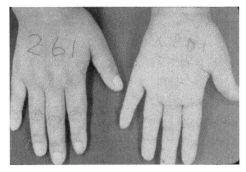

Hand markings of a patient passing through the medical survey stations on the *C.D. Howe*. *X* for X-ray, *P* for physician, *D* for dentist, *I* for immunization. The arrow below the letters means no TB was detected, the individual is free to leave the ship. Courtesy of the Archives of HHS & FHS, Johanna Rabinowitz Fonds.

Overall, these reports give an impression of Northern Affairs people playing catch up with Indian Health and the medical services people, who themselves were staggering under their self-assumed burden of examining every Inuk at least once a year, and finding and evacuating every treatable case of tuberculosis. Undeterred, Willis added work to his program. In 1956 he planned a special Craig Harbour study, which involved members of the medical patrol preparing a detailed report on each family with regard to their "social habits, standards of hygiene, diet and contacts." Also housing, clothing and "degree of adoption of the white man's habits." Moreover, "during this trip four typical cases of tuberculosis of varying age and sex should be selected for special study and comparison."[81]

In 1957, although "the prime purpose of the survey is the ultimate eradication of tuberculosis in the area . . . an attempt is to be made during this survey to accumulate other data . . . Of special interest in this regard are three projects." These were an assessment of Inuit with respect to arteriosclerosis, lots of blood samples for work up in the departmental labs when the party returned from the North, and skin testing on sample groups for trichina and dog tapeworm.[82]

Relentless is the word that comes to mind. But there was something missing in all this. Willis concluded the 1955 report with some remarks on the communication problem: "I feel it is of the utmost importance to set in motion at the earliest opportunity, in co-operation with northern Administration, machinery for sending regular reports on hospital patients to our representatives here. Such messages will quickly break down the barriers of disappointment and distrust that seem to have grown up in the past few years and will pave the way for a badly needed program of health education."[83]

This brings us to consideration of the Inuit experience, that "disappointment and distrust" to which Willis adverts and of which he had seen several instances by the time the *Howe* reached Churchill. At Povungnituk (now Puvirnituq), when he visited the nursing station, he was told that a patient with an abscess of the face had discharged himself on learning that the ship had come in. At Ivujivik, he and Phillips were advised by the local priest that, had Dr. Simpson (the medical officer in '53) been aboard, "I would have taken the Eskimos over the hills before I would let them be examined."[84]

At the time of this remark, the x-ray survey and consequent evacuations had been going on for ten years, having already begun with the *Nascopie* in 1946. There were two sets of grievances. The first had to do with evacuation itself, consisting as it did in a usually sudden and often lengthy (two or three years) exile from home and family to southern Canada, sometimes by plane, sometimes by ship, sometimes by both. The second problem was the lack of communication after evacuation. People in the North received very little news as to the whereabouts or condition of the evacuees.

THREE: EVACUATION

1.

It seems widely believed that Inuit evacuees were coerced or intimidated at the time of evacuation. I have heard an Inuk lobbyist remark that the circumstances were analogous to the residential schools captivity. A newspaper article appearing in 2004 reported that "a medical ship visited the remote village of Inukjuak . . . more than three decades ago.

> A steam-powered behemoth . . . dropped anchor in the frigid waters of Hudson Bay . . .
> A shipboard crane lowered a boat into the water, and soon a doctor arrived on shore with a team of RCMP officers.
> They took the Inuit from their skin tents, gave them dog tags with identification numbers, and loaded them onto a barge. (Graeme Smith)

The occasion of the article was the impending visit of the research vessel *Amundsen*.

In the late summer of 2007 the contingent of forty medical people travelling with forty coast guard personnel on the *Amundsen* attended a plaque unveiling ceremony at Iqaluit in memory of those who were lost to tuberculosis during the days of the evacuations.

> Survey lead Prof. Dr. Grace Egeland of McGill University said the project raised memories of the *C.D. Howe* medical ship in the 1950s . . .

"As we were planning this survey using the ship, the memories of C.D. Howe have come back to people in communities," Egeland told CBC News on Monday. "There's been no closure, no healing, no group ceremony where we can collectively come together to recognize the loss and the tragedy and the suffering of families." ("Nunavut health group to commemorate Inuit TB victims")

An article by Frank Tester, Paule McNicoll and Peter Irniq (Commissioner of Nunavut at the time of its writing) avers that "during the Eastern Arctic Patrol, [Inuit] were often taken aboard ship without consent, X-rayed and sent south – without consent – most often without disembarking to make proper arrangements with their families for the ongoing care of those left behind."

No references or evidence is offered in support of this assertion, even though Tester had read Grygier, who discussed not only the hastiness of departure but also measures taken after 1956 to moderate the hastiness and mitigate its effects. In the matter of evacuation for treatment, there is little in the archival record of officialdom to suggest compulsion, although the question regularly arose. On the other hand, there is much to show that *consent* is not an accurate term for what occurred either. People who were on the *Howe* when diagnosed seem to have "accepted" evacuation, for whatever reasons, more readily than those who were not. There are records of people refusing to go aboard, but I have not found a record of someone aboard insisting on going ashore rather than remain for evacuation. Simpson closed his 1953 report by writing, "Some thought should be given to having all active tuberculosis cases treated. This is a delicate subject and at the present time is probably not feasible. However until all the active cases are under treatment, there will continue to be a spread of new cases."[85]

Simpson had encountered several people who refused to go out for treatment. His remarks were sent on to the head of Arctic Services, with this note under what appear to be the initials of Frank J. G. Cunningham, then director of the Northern Administration and Lands Branch: "Mr. Cantley – for preparation of memo [to] Director re necessity for order making hospitalization mandatory."

James Cantley, however, rejected the proposal:

Although under the Public Health Ordinance of the Northwest Territories the Commissioner is empowered to make regulations for the control of infectious diseases, no regulation has yet been passed . . . While there have been a few cases where Eskimos have refused to go out for treatment, this has been largely due to failure on the part of those dealing with them to explain the reasons for undergoing treatment and for protecting the other members of the community. Arbitrary enforcement of any regulation could create serious difficulties and might do more harm than good. I would say that if we continue to educate the Eskimos on matters of health, there will be little need to enforce treatment.[86]

However, in 1955 Willis was still finding recalcitrant patients.

At Port Harrison a woman with a three-month-old baby was found to have cavities in the left lung. Every attempt to persuade her to come aboard for evacuation failed and she had to be left behind in the hope that, by the time an aircraft was available or McBrien arrived, the Deckers [the woman in charge of the nursing station and her husband, an RCMP constable] could change her mind. This would seem to be an instance where legal power to use force might be needed, but the psychological effects on the other Eskimos of the forcible removal of such cases might only delay our program as a whole and I would certainly recommend that we try health education and persuasion first. At the same time, I see no harm in pressing for the necessary legislation, similar to that provided for in the regulations to the Indian Act.[87]

This seems clear enough. But as the trip continued, the same stubborn reluctance kept reappearing. At Pond Inlet, "in the end five Eskimos were evacuated. One of these . . . a boy of 19, at first refused to come, but Father Daniello and Dr. Schaefer, after spending two hours talking to him and members of his family, finally persuaded him. This part of the work has taken a good deal of our time at each port."[88]

Nor was it only the Inuit who were resisting the doctors. Willis became unhappy with an RCMP staff sergeant, on the ship since Montreal, who "did not help matters at Clyde River. This officer has displayed a gradually increasing lack of sympathy for what we are trying to do. At several settlements he has deliberately set his personnel against us, refusing to allow them to enter into discussion with the Eskimos about the necessity of going out for treatment, taking the stand that there is no legislation to compell [sic] them to go, and failing to see the obvious need, under the circumstances, for practical common sense."[89]

Another two years and H. B. Sabean, medical officer for part of the 1957 patrol, was still wrestling with the same problems:

The legal position is peculiar. On the Quebec coast we had two cases who while they did not refuse evacuation said in effect "but not right now." We had no choice but to leave them behind with recommendations that they be evacuated by other means as soon as possible. Cases seen in the Northwest Territories before our arrival at Pangnirtung could, if necessary, be told that they were to be hospitalized and that if they refused to go "outside" they would have to be taken to the hospital at Pangnirtung. This "threat" was necessary on only a couple of occasions, one case being the old lady from Grise Fjord who refused evacuation in 1955. However, in no case did any of the people approached prefer Pangnirtung to "outside hospitalization." This seems to point at what . . . I had always suspected, that it is not the going "outside" or the hospitalization that they object to as much as it [is] leaving their homes and families.[90]

Thus ten years on, if we date the era of TB evacuation from 1946, the medical authorities continued to treat the issue as one of informed consent to treatment, rather than precautionary quarantine, because compulsion was judged unworkable and self-defeating. Nonetheless it could be done, as it was in at least one region in 1959, though the individuals involved were not Inuit. "The past year there were 4 outstanding cases, who absolutely and point blank refused to come to hospital no matter what the persuasion or advice given by our nurses and the Indian Agent so that we now very reluctantly have had to resort to warrants (Indian Act Form B). I greatly dislike doing this but the disease will never be stamped out unless these active cases are brought under treatment thus removing the source of infection."[91]

According to Johanna van der Woerd, who worked with both Inuit and Cree, Inuit were far more trusting than other First Nations peoples, a difference she thought reflected their shorter experience of Euro-Canadian impositions. "[In] my experience, the Indians didn't trust the whites because they had seen a lot of the whites but they were not always treated by the whites . . . but when an Eskimo came out [by air or train] they'd give themselves over completely and they want to communicate . . . but with the Indians it took a lot longer. Once you knew them, once they trusted you, you were alright but it took quite a while before they really trust you" (personal interview).

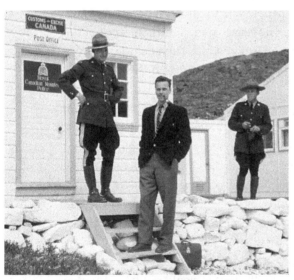

R. A. J. Phillips, touring the Eastern Arctic in 1958. Courtesy of the Archives of HHS & FHS, Johanna Rabinowitz Fonds.

Returning again to Willis in 1955. There was a reluctance to force people, but there was also great ambiguity. "At Lake Harbour six Eskimo patients were taken aboard, not without considerable persuasion and hard work. Most of the second day was spent by members of our party and by Mr. Phillips of Northern Administration and Constable Barr of the RCMP in finding and persuading patients to come aboard for evacuation . . . the immediate diagnosis and evacuation of patients presents serious social welfare and public relations problems, and yet I believe this is the only sensible way to deal with tuberculosis in the North."[92]

Phillips gave a very full account of the difficulties at Lake Harbour and elsewhere, and I reproduce a large part of it here as an example of the intense pressure that was brought to bear on people, and the futility of attempting to distinguish between consent and coercion in the circumstances surrounding evacuation.

> This relationship between the local R.C.M.P. and other Government agencies, which reaches something short of warmhearted [*sic*] co-operation, was again evident in the most difficult problem we had in Lake Harbour, the evacuation of [Jane] and her relatives. This woman was discovered last year to have a most serious case of T.B. in a highly infectious stage. An x-ray confirmed that her husband of six months now also was seriously infected. Dr. Willis regarded the evacuation of both as a matter of the highest importance, not only to the lives of these two people but for the safety of the whole community. If they were not evacuated, the whole work of the survey party would be undermined and Tuberculosis, far from being eliminated, might gain new strength in the population of 275.
>
> Unfortunately, [Jane] was reluctant to come out. On our first night, Miss Anerodluk, accompanied by Dr. Willis, tried long to persuade her. At one point she acquiesced but then disappeared. Her husband did come to the ship. The next morning, therefore, one of our principal tasks in Lake Harbour was to persuade this woman to come out. If she had gone over the hills as was reported, we were prepared even to use the helicopter to talk to her again. The R.C.M.P., however, refused to have anything to do with her evacuation; S/Sgt. Kearney told Dr. Willis that it would not be in keeping with the dignity of the Force to go chasing an Eskimo woman through the hills.

Next morning I flew over to the R.C.M.P. to talk the problem over with them. I told S/Sgt. Kearney and Constable Barr that I was fully aware of the lack of legislation. We have a problem here that regulations did not cover. One human life was immediately at stake as well as the health of the community and possibly the lives of others in it. How could we persuade this patient to come and be treated?

I was told that there was no law, that there should be a law, and that if National Health and Welfare and we had not been so stupid there would have been a law by now. This was a consequence of our own policies. I repeated that I knew the legal position, that we were now facing a practical problem and I wished to draw on their experience and help in order to solve it. Could any means be found for getting this woman to the ship? I was informed that Eskimos were full Canadian citizens and that you cannot herd them about. I said that she was living with 274 other full Canadian citizens and that nowhere else in Canada would stand idly by while these other citizens were exposed to the intimate danger in which they also now lived. I was told that it was against Regulations, that they would not touch the case. (Their attitude to our problem was indicated even before this conversation by Barr's conspicuous absence from the camp, that is from the people for whom he is responsible, while our staff, all strangers to the woman, was making all the efforts to persuade her to come out. Of course, Barr's establishment was being inspected by S/Sgt. Kearney at the time, and priority of business has many interpretations.) I was told that any action by the Police would be contrary to all principles on which the Force was founded. I said that I could not agree that it would be contrary to all the principles of the Force – to the human principle. There was nothing in the Regulations. Did I intend to allow myself open to a charge of kidnapping? I said that I had not come to suggest kidnapping but to ask the Police to help talk to the woman. Would they

NOBODY HERE WILL HARM YOU

do so? They were sorry, but they were very busy: anyway, this was Health and Welfare's problem, not the Police's . . .

From this depressing tale a happy end emerges: the woman and her husband came aboard. Mr. Manning and Miss Anerodluk had a series of conversations with the woman, using every technique of persuasion – a last talk between Mr. Manning and the patient lasted over two hours. I cannot speak too highly either of the service which Mr. Manning performed in this case or his skill in carrying it out.[93]

It may be that Lake Harbour people were remembering an earlier incident, cited by Bishop Marsh in a bitter letter of February 1954 to Gordon Robertson. "I only wish that you might have seen, as I have seen at Lake Harbour, Eskimo children being wrested without notice from their mother and fathers, from their families, placed on a ship and taken to the unknown outside. The policeman who was forced to do it was almost in tears."[94] Phillips does not mention this incident, and Marsh was much given to drama, but the administrator does allow that

the medical procedure in the past was the subject of criticism and even contempt. Public relations with the Eskimos had been badly handled and, as a consequence, it was difficult to persuade the T.B. patients to leave for the outside. There had been glib promises of early return, promises which Government officials might have known could not be kept. There had been carelessness in follow up. For instance, last year the doctor had taken away a pair of broken glasses, the wearer's only pair, to have a replacement made. Nothing further was heard of them and Dr. Willis was told nothing about them.[95]

In addition to the declining credibility of Euro-Canadian authority, the length of the absences and the poor communication were no doubt adding to the hesitations of people urged to go out. One of the repatriates on the *Howe* in 1955 with Phillips and Willis was Kenojuak Ashevak, who had been at Parc Savard since 1952. In the winter of 1951, when she was told by Mounties travelling between Cape Dorset and Lake Harbour that her x-ray was positive, she refused to be taken out until she had seen her husband, who was away. Her newborn she gave up for adoption before leaving. While she was in southern Canada, her other two children died. Rare letters were all the contact she had with home. Stories like this, as they became known in northern communities, would alone be enough to engender resistance to evacuation.

Phillips's problems with that resistance were just beginning. At Clyde River, he wrote,

> The medical survey began about midnight with all the Health and Welfare staff and five people from other Departments assisting. Sixty-two people were examined by shortly after 5:00 a.m. The staff then went to bed to be ready to begin again at 10:00 a.m. As usual, the Eskimos were not on hand but anticipating this problem I flew ashore beforehand to help round them up.
>
> The R.C.M.P. once again offered no assistance whatsoever, preferring to stay as far as possible from the whole operation . . . By morning, however, it was time to call in the R.C.M.P. to see where the missing 31 were . . . I therefore flew over to Cape Christian and explained to Staff Sergeant and Constable Marshall that I would like Constable Marshall's help in identifying the remaining 31 Eskimos and in finding four or five people who required treatment in the south. I did not raise any question of persuading people to go south, asking only for help in finding people within the community. Constable Marshall was anxious to get an easy form of transportation to Clyde River and he agreed to come, but my invitation was an occasion for Staff Sergeant Kearney to tell Marshall in my presence that he was to have nothing to do with the evacuation, that it was a matter for the doctors. I said gently to him that I thought that it was a matter for all of us servants of the Government. The Staff Sergeant did not agree and went on to instruct Marshall that he might say

that it was a good thing for T.B. patients to go to hospital but if they showed any reluctance he was to have no further conversation with them. The time was too short to convert the Staff Sergeant and so I climbed into the plane asking Marshall if he would come along to help us at least find the other 30 people. Staff Sergeant Kearney then called Marshall back for a further three or four minutes of conversation alone. Mr Marshall got in the plane and I asked him, "Well, were you getting your last minute instructions to give no assistance to the medical party or the Patrol?" "Yes," Constable Marshall replied frankly.

When we arrived at Clyde River, Marshall said that he was unable to speak to the Eskimos and he wanted Reverend [Tom] Daulby, a passenger on the "C.D. Howe" enroute to Pond Inlet, to do it for him . . . [Manning has evidently left the ship, though Phillips does not indicate when or where.] We sent for Mr. Daulby with some reluctance; he was apparently the only person who could communicate with the Eskimos in the absence of Miss Anerodluk who was fully occupied in the medical quarters [i.e., the patrol has come to a village of 84 inhabitants with one Inuktitut speaker]. Mr Daulby was of the greatest assistance and thanks largely to his efforts not only did we round up 85% of all the residents of Clyde River but we persuaded every patient to accept treatment outside . . .

When I mentioned the names of two of the seriously infected cases, Marshall and Kearney asked if we really had to take these people because their absence would create relief problems. Later, when Mr. Daulby persuaded the patients to go out for treatments, Staff Sergeant Kearney sent a message saying that the R.C.M.P. would give no relief to any of the dependents without written instructions from the Department of Northern Affairs. I said that I was quite agreeable to authorizing relief and would accept his recommendations on the amount. He said that it was not up to the R.C.M.P. to advise, that Northern Affairs made its own rules and it was up to Northern Affairs to apply them. He told me that I should get my departmental instructions out and organize the relief before the ship pulled out.

As Staff Sergeant Kearney was well aware, time was desperately short and everyone aboard had far more to do than consult relief regulations. Even Marshall thought this was pretty silly pettifoggery and when I asked him if he could not give one full ration to each member of the families involved, cutting it if meat became available, he agreed. I therefore had an authorization to this effect typed. Marshall pocketed it without bothering to read it.

The Staff Sergeant wasted our time in other irritating little ways while we were trying hard to finish our work on time, interrupting a meeting to announce that a girl was in tears, that we could not leave her bereft of parents and that we had better do something about it. After Dr. Willis and I had succeeded in finding Mr. Daulby and the girl we found that there was no question of evacuation of her or any relative and that the reason for the tears was as obscure as in any woman.[96]

This is poor, and nobody was being done justice. The child was certainly upset about something, so there may have been some connection between her and an evacuee that Daulby did not uncover. Or she may simply have been upset to see that others were. In any case, the situation in itself was enough to alarm anyone exposed to it. Phillips and Willis had landed here, rounded up everyone they could, stampeded eight onto the boat and, despite the fact that the itinerary was decided in Ottawa months before, no arrangement whatever had been made for easing the distress or assuring the sustenance of those who may be left behind without the usual providers. Several pages after this account of the conflicts with Kearney, Phillips wrote that

the father of the boy who urgently required medical attention to save his sight adamantly refused to let his son go out. Four years ago they had taken another son on the promise he would be back in a year. He is still outside and the news from him is scanty and infrequent. This year absolutely no promises are being made. We can however, hope that beginning next year most of the T.B. cases will have had only one year to develop and the length of treatment will therefore tend to be shorter. Nevertheless, it remains a puzzling and discouraging fact that the healing of lesions in Eskimos requires, on the average, about double the time as in other patients.[97]

From this, it can be inferred that resistance may have been proportionate to the numbers already evacuated. According to P. G. Nixon, during the whole period about seventy percent of Clyde River adults went out. Obviously, the memory of Clyde River must be consulted to learn why resistance was so strong there. The written record can suggest possibilities, but the Inuit account is needed to confirm or deny these speculations.

The medical information claimed here by Phillips is suspect as is much else, but generally the impression given is that Clyde River was simply beyond the resources of the patrol. Phillips felt obliged by his conspicuous position to demonstrate energy and authority, to act with or without understanding. At Pond Inlet, the problems continued: "Dr. Willis and I arranged to fly in an hour before the ship dropped anchor to organize the first movement of people from ashore. The Captain was naturally quite happy with this arrangement for it was primarily designed to help us complete the survey by the time his cargo was unloaded and so forestall any delay in departure. We struck a snag, however. Staff Sergeant Kearney objected to the Doctor and me going ashore before him."[98]

Some back and forth ensued, and Phillips prevailed, because he had previously secured a monopoly on the helicopter. Here is a literal example of how technological advances were the politics of this period in the North, in that it allowed the Canadian State to take hold of territories it could previously reach but not hold. In the conclusions he attached to his report, Phillips gave a section to the helicopter. He explained how he came to an arrangement with the captain to have the fullest possible use of the machine, originally intended by the Department of Transport primarily for ice patrol. "For my part I would take responsibility for assigning the helicopter to members of the Patrol. No members of the Patrol were to approach him for its use and he would give none of them authority to use it."[99] Phillips carried Ottawa's flag into every port ahead of the *Howe*, and visited places the *Howe* had to bypass because of fog or ice. On this day at Pond Inlet, he used it to neutralize Kearney's control over his own forces. Consequently,

> the local R.C.M.P. were very helpful in the organization of the medical survey. Partly this was because Corporal Moodie and Constable Cooley were themselves capable and sympathetic; partly also the doctor and I were forced to conclude that they were helpful because we had enlisted their support before Staff Sergeant Kearney was able to order them to have nothing to do with the survey. Nevertheless on the morning following our arrival he made a speech to his men in the presence of Dr. Willis, Mr. Ross and Miss MacArthur in which he said that they were to have no part in persuading the people to have medical examinations let alone accepting treatment in the south if they had T.B. He also criticized Northern Affairs for not having Miss Anerodluk on shore to round up the Eskimos, ignoring the fact that she was already doing two jobs in the sick bay area in the course of the medical examinations. Staff Sergeant Kearney's instructions on this occasion came too late to hamper seriously the operation and even after it both Moodie and Cooley were co-operative. Ninety people were examined and five were found to be positive. There was no difficulty in persuading them to go out.[100]

It is hard to believe that there was no difficulty, but whatever the circumstances, in Willis's day, when a number of Euro-Canadians – including a policeman, whose authority in Arctic hamlets was augmented by his sharing control of patronage (and sometimes credit and family allowance payments) with the local HBC man and any resident clerics – approached an Inuk and began to insist upon something, the usual meaning of *consent* no longer applied. Presumably this was in part what troubled the balky RCMP sergeant who so exasperated Willis and Phillips.

As Phillips tells it, his overriding concern was to protect the non-tuberculous ("the innocent" as he called them), from those who were infected and contagious by removing the latter from the community to whom they posed "an intimate danger." In recommending legislation, in order to save "the innocent," he remarked, "This year we have left in the country people with serious cases of tuberculosis, some with small children, who are almost bound to contract it before the ship comes again. To leave these people to their fate is not treating them as first class citizens. If we are not concerned with answering to ourselves for what we are doing then we might be moved by consideration of how we would answer to the public if the present state of affairs should ever become a matter of general criticism and controversy."[101]

This concern was reinforced by reports such as he had at Port Harrison, that a certain Inuk who had been told two years running of the need to accept evacuation and had refused, had now lost two of his children to tuberculous meningitis. Not an outcome that would please Kearney or anyone, so what was Kearney's problem? Instead of taking a brief from him, as Phillips did from anything that moved in every port of call, the Officer in Charge decided to contest with him in order to assert the nascent supremacy of Northern Affairs.

In 1955 Health and Welfare was in its tenth year of evacuations. Moreover, Phillips believed that in that time it had been learned that Inuit lesions took twice as long to heal as those of Euro-Canadians. But he remained oblivious, or at least silent, on the lack, ten years on, of any organization for the welfare of those left behind by evacuees. The confrontations he described evidently still packed a punch for him. These passages appear to have been written in response to another version of events he imagined was in preparation or already in circulation. He tells the story very vividly, and displays the ferocious indignation that arises whenever one recognizes that one's opponent may be in the right. However, this recognition usually leads also, in fairly short order, to concessions, which are absent here. The problem that Kearney was trying to drive home to the boss at Clyde River is not even acknowledged, not in the main text of the report or in the lengthy conclusions. Phillips placed great emphasis on the need for sustained and frequent communications between the hospitalized and their homes, but did not mention advance preparation for evacuation or measures to ease the emotional toll of departure. Surely there is something wrong here. The absence needs an explanation. Phillips was too humane and thoughtful a man – Willis likewise – not to see that removing people from home so very abruptly would cause serious problems. It is like tugging a strand out of a tapestry. Removing partners from a semi-nomadic group will impair its functioning. But he committed not a word to paper on the subject. Willis, however, did acknowledge the problems in a report: "As indicated in my initial weekly report, the immediate diagnosis and evacuation of patients presents serious social welfare and public relations problems, and yet I believe this is the only sensible way to deal with tuberculosis in the North. There have been several individual cases which have brought this forcibly to our attention."[102]

The following year saw the hiring of Walter Rudnicki to set up a welfare branch. This was a tacit vindication of Kearney, but driven by whom? If it was not Phillips, was it Willis? Or perhaps Sivertz, who already in 1954 had said, "In my opinion, this department needs to operate what amounts to a medical social welfare service which will bring us into close co-operation with Indian Health Services in respect to the whole medical program,"[103] and was finally able to follow through? Just to show the improbable variety of human affairs, it was possible for evacuation to not only be accepted but even sought. Margery Hinds encountered a case while at her Cape Dorset posting:

> One of my worst and really frightening times concerned a girl whose stepfather was insisting on having sexual intercourse with her. The girl's mother also came to me to ask my help in trying to get the girl away, even though the girl was with her stepfather's baby. Apparently the mother had already tried to enlist the help of . . . the chief Catechist and most important camp leader. She had also asked the R.C. Missionary although the family was not R.C. . . . The woman thought that at ship

time maybe the medical team would find the girl had T.B. and would be taken "outside." If not, perhaps in this special case, the doctors would pretend that something was wrong and that the girl could be taken away. I suggested this to the doctor but he objected . . . The policy decision was that the girl be taken out by the R.C.M.P. and taken to her relatives at Frobisher Bay which is what happened. (quoted in Macpherson, 129)

Finally, there was in fact a standard form of consent, titled Agreement to Accept Medical and Surgical Treatment, used on the *Howe* from 1957, and perhaps earlier: "I, the undersigned, hereby agree to accept medical treatment. I declare that I am the person herein identified, and that I am unable to pay for adequate treatment otherwise. I authorize to be performed on my person whatever examination, treatment, or operation is indicated in the opinion of the medical authorities and I undertake to co-operate fully in all measures to maintain treatment and discipline."[104]

To this was appended a witness statement: "I, the undersigned, state that the above declaration has been interpreted to the signee, that he has expressed acknowledgement of the understanding of its content and has, in my presence, affixed his signature thereto."[105] Below, the same formulae were repeated for guardians.

It is difficult to construe this as anything other than ceremony. *Any* operation?

Presumably this was meant to apply in the immediate circumstance of an examination and any on-the-spot treatment given. What, if anything, was done in the event of a diagnosis of active tuberculosis, and all that followed, seems to have been in the hands of the interpreters. Consent to evacuation certainly implies consent to treatment, but to what treatment, and with what explanations? To chemotherapy, yes, but to possible allergic reactions? To surgery, with possible complications? Joanasie Salamonie of Cape Dorset told Pat Grygier that while he was at Parc Savard he thought that the doctors were practising on him – an indication that there was not a great deal of consultation with the recipient about the nature of his treatment and the choices involved (Grygier, 115).

From all this we may conclude that evacuation was first of all a quarantine procedure, a fact somewhat obscured by the circumstance that the best quality of treatment required expatriation, and confused further by the circumstance that isolation of the infected could not occur on the ship, because no real provision had been made to effect it when the *Howe* was built. The conundrum faced by would-be imposers of quarantine was, which is better? To enforce removal and isolation of the infectious and risk wide non-compliance when news of enforcement spreads, or to take a more relaxed approach, with potentially the same result: more infection? Given the room available for anyone who wished to run, the EAP doctors had to give Inuit patients a choice. They could have attempted to enforce quarantine once the patient was essentially trapped on the boat, but this would simply have deterred people from coming aboard the *Howe* or her sister vessels at all, and risked still further medical complications.

On the other hand, for many years the Inuit had no choice other than evacuation or no treatment whatsoever, which, given the nature of the active disease, amounts to no choice.

Once in hospital, with nothing to be done, the northerners gave over and co-operated entirely, and afterwards expressed appreciation for their cure. Getting there however (and back) was another matter, especially if one came out on the boat. This could be a very uncomfortable and tedious voyage.

Bob Williamson recalled conditions aboard the *Howe* in 1953/54 for Alexandra Grygier: "The ship was deep in misery. It was terrible because it was the ship which carried the Inuit away from their homes to the sanatoria in the south. And they were herded together in the foc'sle, in the hold of the ship in three-tiered bunks, mass fed, mass accommodated. In the stormy seas they were sick, they were terrified, they were demoralized. They were frightened of what was happening to them, of what was likely to happen to them" (quoted in Grygier, 86).

In 1957 Sabean reported that from Churchill on it was like this:

We carried on an average of fifty transients at all times; the actual number varied and at times there were about ninety people jammed into the Eskimo Quarters and Sick Bay area. This was perhaps partly my fault as perhaps I should have insisted that we accept fewer repatriates for transit; it was felt however, that to leave people in Churchill, for example, who were destined for Howe ports of call would be the greater of two evils . . . Northern Affairs took an active interest and accepted a good deal of responsibility for conditions in the Eskimo Quarters . . . Their program for on the spot needle work for the women and carving for the men was helpful as at least in some cases it helped to keep up the moral [*sic*] of the people in transit . . . The captain was quite worried and somewhat unsatisfied with conditions in the Eskimo quarters . . . The toilets were forever being plugged, broken and dirtied; drainage tanks which stored effluent from sinks were frequently overflowing onto the floors; bunks being broken from the walls; etc. These things received prompt attention from the ship's crew.[106]

The plane was not so hot either. Sarah Saimaiyuk of Pangnirtung went out by float plane to Moose Factory: "During the flight we got very thirsty and we were frightened. My little sister, who was only a baby then, started crying. I was so thirsty that my mouth got very dry, and we couldn't tell the qallunaat [non-Inuit] who were with us, because we didn't speak their language. Although I knew the word for water in English, I didn't say anything, thinking there was no water in the airplane. I was so frightened of the qallunaat" (Saimaiyuk and Saimaiyuk, 21).

From Moose Factory she went on by train to Mountain San. On arrival at the hospital, she was separated from her sister. All this without interpreters until she met patients from Puvirnituq at the hospital who could speak both languages, but whose dialect was so removed from her own that she could not at first understand.

Complaints, however, were not about the journey but rather about the abruptness of evacuation and the worry about those left behind, and about the paucity of communication between the North and the evacuees.

2.

Leo Manning, an old Arctic hand and proficient Inuktitut speaker who had served the HBC in Labrador, as well as in the Eastern and Western Arctic, was recruited to government service in 1952. In the late winter of the following year, he was looking in on Inuit patients in Quebec hospitals and writing his boss, James Cantley, to tell what he had found: "I left Ottawa on Monday, February 23rd at 7:40 a.m. and arrived in Montreal at 11 a.m. In the afternoon, Mr J.V. Jacobsen of the Education Branch and I set out for Sacred Heart Hospital at Caughnawaga [Kahnawake]. Due to a misunderstanding on the part of the taxi driver, we were taken to Sacred Heart Hospital at Cartierville. Upon making inquires there; it was found that there were two Eskimo patients in the hospital of which we had no record."[107]

This was inexact. Cartierville does indeed appear on a list of "hospitals where there are Eskimo patients" prepared by Cantley on February 13, ten days prior to Manning's visit. Cantley made the list for Simpson, who had provided Cantley with a roll of Inuit evacuees in southern Canada. But things were not in good order.

> Although the greatest concentration of Eskimo patients is at Parc Savard and Charles Camsell from which we receive reports, it would be of great assistance to us if we could receive quarterly reports, in the regular form, from all Hospitals [there were twenty at this point] where Eskimos are being treated ... In view of the large numbers coming out now for treatment, we find that it is very necessary to have up-to-date information on them. We are interested not only their progress but also in knowing what provision, if any, we must make from time to time for the care of their dependents, where there are any. We also receive frequent inquiries from the field as to the location of patients and the progress they are making.[108]

In other words, the Indian Health Services and its medical patrol had gotten well ahead of itself. Up to February 1953 at least, it seems no one had given much attention to establishing lines of communication between patients and their communities – and authorities began to feel the lack of information. The problem was not new, but already fixed and chronic in 1950, when J. C. Osborne was medical officer in charge on the *Howe*, and urgently recommended the following:

> That in future some person or persons [be] made responsible for following up those Eskimo patients who are evacuated to hospitals outside from the Eastern Arctic, and submitting by radio-telegram every few months to the post from which the patient has come a progress report on each case. So far as I have been able to tell, this is a responsibility which has in the past been entirely neglected. The Eskimo do not on the whole object to having their loved ones taken from them on the advice of the white man, but they do resent not hearing any news of these evacuees for months or even years on end. Repeatedly during the trip I was asked questions about the health and whereabouts of patients who had been evacuated months or even years previously, and about whom no word of information had ever reached the relatives . . . Many of these people were not even aware as to whether their next of kin were alive or dead . . . All that is required is for some one person to keep track of all these cases and send out every two or three months by radio or mail a bulletin to the home of the patient in question. I cannot stress too strongly the importance of taking action of this recommendation. It is indeed probably the most important of all the recommendations which I have made.[109]

In February 1953, Leo Manning was partially fulfilling the role urged by Osborne, but by 1955 Manning was hard at work helping Willis and Phillips persuade people to come out. So the communications deficit persisted, and if Manning was dealing with the other problem – arranging for the care of the dependents of evacuees, young or old – no one was reporting that activity. Manning continued to offer himself, and be accepted, as an intermediary and messenger until his death in 1958, and forty or so of the letters he received in 1956 from Inuit patients and their kin seeking assistance or information have been discussed in detail by Frank Tester, Paule McNicoll and Peter Irniq (121–40).[110]

There was also the question as to what all these expatriated and demobilized patients (in 1953, there were one hundred four of them at Parc Savard alone) might actually *do* all day. The women were making socks and mittens, and the men, woodcarvings. "There is a rumour," Manning reported, "that a handicraft technician was to visit the hospital in early April to study the situation and to see what could be done. Dr. Labrecque informed me that there would be no objection to the natives using Narwhal tusks."[111] The impending technician was probably sculptor Harold Pfeiffer, whose brother was in fact a doctor at the hospital. Among the patients languishing at Savard at that time was Kenojuak Ashevak, who began her artistic career there. This gap in services was not new either, but had been clearly recognized in 1952 at a meeting of the Eskimo Affairs Committee, during which the committee was asked to approve a request for $6,700 to hire two welfare teachers. One would join the staff at the Charles Camsell, the second would go to Parc Savard.[112]

The communication problem was twofold: Individuals needed to be reconnected with people awaiting them back home, and people in the North needed to be given some vague idea of what went on in southern hospitals they had never seen. Accordingly, as Sivertz reported from the *Howe* during the 1954 tour, "The Welfare teacher at Parc Savard had made several reels of talk on a tape recorder, mostly messages from Eskimos in hospital addressed to friends in the north. These were listened to with great interest by the Eskimos at several places and some reels of reply were made and mailed to Quebec."[113]

Mailed. Does this mean placed in a bag for eventual delivery by the *Howe* many weeks later? Or does it mean dispatched on the next likely plane? However it may have been, the inference is that the means and lines of communication existed, but that there was still no one who had been made responsible for organizing things.

This is near the heart of the problem. In the same document, Sivertz, chief of Arctic services and officer in charge of the EAP, called his position "anomalous."

> The Captain follows precedents of long standing in arranging, with little or no consultations, such things as times of arrival and departure, route, speed, communications, changes in itinerary, etc. The medical work similarly is carried on as a separate operation with, as a rule, no discussion of the various procedures, some of which have aspects that touch the responsibilities of this department . . . I did not have a very good opportunity to assess the work that was done by this group because at a fairly early stage of the voyage the doctor in charge told me that he felt the Department of National Health and Welfare was solely responsible for the medical program and that it was therefore not the business of my department. I do not think he was correct but there was no object in discussing the matter further if this was his conviction in the light of several years experience in the Eastern Arctic Patrol.[114]

In fact, both the Department of Transport captain and the Indian Health Services personnel were not acquitting themselves very well. The *Howe* was in very poor order, and IHS was reaching about a third of those it wished to serve, and still failing to maintain contacts between evacuees and their home communities. Sivertz continued, "In my opinion, this department needs to operate what amounts to a medical social welfare service which will bring us into close co-operation with Indian Health Services in respect of the whole medical program."[115]

Later that year, in a letter to Margery Hinds at Cape Dorset hastily composed on the last day for the Christmas airdrop (November 26), Sivertz said that he had

> asked for the appointment of a professional person in the field of social welfare to advise us and to organize better means of

keeping in touch with people who are out in hospital or away from their families in other ways.

This time next year I hope to see news of everybody on the outside transmitted to the north in the Christmas air drop. This year our staff is still far too thin and our funds insufficient to visit the hospitals often enough for this purpose. There is a very great deal of development in many places in the north and we are hard put to it to keep up.[116]

The following summer, Sivertz urged that Health and Welfare work with Northern Administration to set up regular reporting from southern hospitals to the North. By December 1955 George Rudnicki had been hired for social welfare along with a staff of two: Leo Manning and Paulette Anerodluk (Grygier, 81).

Willis's team had shown some film from the Mountain San during the 1955 tour, and the collection of messages to be brought south was improved also. In June, just before the ship was to depart Montreal, the superintendent of education wrote an urgent letter asking for the purchase of a better tape recorder:

As you are aware, on the Eastern Arctic Patrol, messages are recorded from relatives and friends of patients hospitalized at points outside of the Northwest Territories . . . At the present time a Recordio Tape Recorder is used for this purpose. This machine is fairly large and operates on 110 Volt, 60 cycle Alternating Current and can only be used where there is an adequate source of power. In order to record messages from Eskimos in their own homes or out in the open in the summer time, the ideal recording device would be portable . . . operated from batteries. There is only one such machine on the market; it is a MOHAWK Midgetape – priced at $229.50 . . . It would be appreciated if you would arrange to have this recording device purchased immediately without the usual procedure of submitting a requisition and sent with [Phillips] on the ship for use by Mr. E. N. Grantham.[117]

Five years and hundreds of evacuations after Osborne's recommendation, the whereabouts of individuals who had been evacuated was still vague to those back home. Sarah Saimaiyuk, in a 1990 account, said, "In the residence [at Moose Factory] I saw a wooden bed that had been used by a patient coming back from Hamilton. On it he had written the names of all the patients, and messages. That's how I learned I was going to Hamilton" (Saimaiyuk and Saimaiyuk, 22).

After Rudnicki's hiring, both communications and pre-evacuation arrangements improved, but not instantly. In 1957 he sent Ruth Banffy on the *Howe* to appraise the situation.[118] Banffy was succeeded by Betty Marwood the following year, and Marwood stayed in the job until 1964. According to Grygier, she was able, starting in 1959, to make three important changes to the EAP survey procedure. First, she became the link between the doctors and those patients who were slated for evacuation. It was she who conveyed the bad news, and who took the time to discuss the situation and solve any problems. Second, she convinced the doctors to let patients leave the ship to put their affairs in order and collect whatever they might wish to bring out with them. Third, she convinced the Department of Transport that the ship must wait on the completion of her work, even if all supply and survey work were already done. She also ensured that photographs were taken of the outgoing patient with their family, so that the patient would have this token while in southern Canada (Grygier, 101).[119]

The question arises, why had the doctors, who had been pulling people outside in ever-increasing numbers for ten years, not previously organized these rather obvious services?

3.

The Department of Health and Welfare, with P. E. Moore in charge, took over the medical responsibilities previously discharged by the Indian Affairs branch of the Department of Mines and Resources on November 1, 1945.

During that year, three doctors worked for the EAP on the *N.B. McLean* and the *Nascopie*. On their return these men had a lot to say. They rejected outside sanatorium treatment for Inuit, recommending instead a chain of hospitals and nursing stations to serve TB patients and all others together, and warned of the danger of a smallpox epidemic warranting quick precautionary vaccinations of whites and Inuit alike. They had much else to advise and urge, and they did not confine themselves to immediate medical concerns.

The physician on the *McLean*, Dr. R. C. Hastings, was especially wide-ranging in his brief, noting that, "Unfortunately the native is a deaf-mute politically and so far removed geographically that he is well beyond the scope of social and welfare agencies."[120] Infant mortality was very high. Since the greatest need was infant and maternal care (not tuberculosis, whose incidence and severity remained to be evaluated) he proposed essentially a system of visiting doctors, preferably women, operating from coasting boats, to address this problem urgently. Later, "native girls" should be trained up as nurses – perhaps at existing facilities at North West River, NL, or Cartwright, NL. This and much else was recorded in Section IV of his report, "Native Health and Welfare." Section V focused on "Native Economy and Social Sciences," including education. Not yet content, he went on to a Section VI, "The Administration of Native Affairs."

Most of what Hastings advanced did eventually occur – but he was certainly very early, and his presumption drew a rebuke from Roy A. Gibson, the deputy minister of the territories, who felt it necessary to remind Moore that "any comment of Dr. Hastings which relates to other than medical matters and hospitalization is looked upon as something within the purview of the Bureau of Northwest Territories and Yukon Affairs and we will deal with it here."[121] He continued on in the same vein for a couple of pages. "It is indeed unfortunate that when Dr. Hastings wished to make such far-reaching recommendations he apparently did not consider it worth his while to discuss his ideas with the officers of the Bureau of Northwest Territories and Yukon Affairs . . . As it turns out he has made errors which indicate that he lacks sufficient knowledge of the subjects which he has attempted to discuss."[122] Finally, the administration had made the best of the resources provided. Now that the "control of medical matters" had been transferred, and more money was likely forthcoming, better days lay ahead.

The following year, the first good picture of the tuberculosis situation was obtained by means of portable x-ray equipment supplied to the EAP on the *Nascopie*. With about twenty-two percent of the total population of six thousand surveyed during the 1946 patrol, impression and conjecture were replaced by factual knowledge. Previously, medical concern had hesitated among several priorities. Tuberculosis, present and evidently burdensome but indistinct, was one. The others were diseases of the eye, onerous and very consequential for people who must hunt and sew to live; the steep rate of infant mortality; and the danger of sudden, intense epidemics when small pockets of the population were exposed to new pathogens carried in by the evermore frequent visitors from far outside. (A 1945 outbreak of gastroenteritis, later identified as typhoid fever, swelled the deaths on West Baffin to forty-five in a six-month period.[123]) The combination of case-finding technology, improved transportation and organization, along with the imperative of isolation to break contagion, the introduction of lastingly effective chemotherapy and the freeing up of space and personnel suggested a campaign of evacuation. Also entering the mix was fear of the emergence of a resistant strain of the bug, and fear of the attentions of urgent, unsubtle newspapers. The press was a new player, and while the HBC's *Beaver* and Phillip's *North/Nord* were anodyne if useful house organs, both devoted to maintaining esprit de corps, there were other publications that would ask hard questions if aroused.[124]

The best discussion of Health and Welfare's accession to control over medical matters, of the tensions between it and other agencies active in the North, and of the contradictory policies that blunted initiative within Northern Affairs is P. G. Nixon's "Early Administrative Developments in Fighting Tuberculosis among Canadian Inuit: Bringing State Institutions Back In." He shows how the doctors gained control of the administration of health and contrasts that department – a stable, comparatively well-funded bureaucracy – with its ever-shifting, politically confused counterpart on the administrative side. The difference comes down to this: Health and Welfare had narrow purposes, clearly defined, and therefore was able to develop plans and execute them. Northern Affairs, even after the reorganization that brought in Phillips and Sivertz, then Snowden and Rudnicki, was uncertain as to its purposes, which were initially contradictory anyway, and then uncertain as to how or whether the ultimate goal – economic independence – could be reached. Back in Ottawa after the 1955 excursion on the *Howe*, while composing his account, Phillips found himself envying Willis: "He knows just where he is going and if he gets sufficient support he will achieve his objectives, the book will be closed and he can turn to some other task. His job is easy because the problems are measurable. He can with relative ease diagnose the illness and organize the medicine or the surgery to cure it. It is merely a matter of time and distance. The problem with which he deals is almost entirely physical and it requires only effective organization."[125]

Unhappily this seems to have been Willis's view as well, and also Moore's during the years prior to the establishment of Northern Health Services in 1954. How can the emphasis on the physical and measurable to the neglect of all else on the part of physicians who certainly knew better and said so all the time be explained? How had "medical matters" become so narrowly defined? Nixon stops at this: "On the big issues of southern hospitalization and northern rehabilitation centres, . . . [the] 'medical view' did prevail." That is, evacuation was preferred and rehab centres were delayed and minimized, because some of the doctors in charge – notably Harry A. Procter, Moore's deputy – felt that in many cases it would be better for the ex-TB patient to remain in southern Canada permanently. This prevalence of the medical view, however, Nixon continues, "was not a foregone conclusion . . . and was determined at least in part by internal state processes including the restrictive . . . role northern administration played regarding Inuit Health Policy, and their lack of more general institutional strength and political support *at this point in time* relative to the physicians of Health and Welfare" (italics original; Nixon, "Early Administrative Developments," 80).

This brings us to is the heart of the problem: why did the physicians attend to what they attended to, and neglect what they neglected? The choice for evacuation has been dealt with; it remains to consider the neglect of social welfare accommodation for those left behind, and the failure to assure communications. There was disagreement within Health and Welfare, as well as between that department and the various permutations of northern administration. The doctors recruited to the annual EAP were mostly occasional, who went along once or twice – though many went twice. They reported and recommended, but were not permanently present to influence the course of things. (There were exceptions, those who went to the nursing stations – Sabean to Pangnirtung, Schaefer to Aklavik and later to Pangnirtung.) The lack of responsiveness must be ascribed to Moore and his deputies – Procter and Willis. Although things changed under Willis, the social welfare changes seem not to have occurred *through* him, but rather through Sivertz, or perhaps Phillips.

Hastings (and also the other doctors of the 1945 patrol) pronounced too firmly on too little experience, but the inclusiveness of his perspective was certainly warranted, and was in fact the mode of the day. The determinants of health, good or ill, are broad. But the expression of this view was treated as an act of trespass. So the doctors were in charge, fine, but much of what conditioned health was placed off limits to them. Their energies were focused on the TB survey and on vaccination – mechanical procedures that were necessary, but mechanical nonetheless – and on the grand goal of the eradication of certain diseases, to the exclusion of other desiderata for well being. As more and more people were brought out and eventually discharged from treatment, the department was obliged to edge back into the territory it had surrendered to administration, and began to discuss the placing of rehabilitation centres in the North. In the spring of 1953, for example, at the second meeting of the Committee on Eskimo Affairs, Moore reported that five hundred Inuit were in hospital during 1952. There was a single rehabilitation centre at Driftpile, AB, that could accommodate six persons. Something similar was planned for Frobisher Bay. The deputy minister, Major-General Hugh A. Young, felt that a facility at Aklavik, where a vocational school was under construction, might be a good idea. Moore concurred. However, since the Inuit population was now likely to grow until it exceeded the carrying capacity of the region, he wished to acquire from the United Church at Edmonton a farm and school "which could be used to fit Eskimos for integration into the Canadian economy, either in the Arctic or in the South."[126]

But still nothing was contemplated in the way of pre-habilitation, so to speak, until 1956 or 1957. This lacuna is puzzling: not only socially disturbing, but medically unsound. That is, from within the perspective of the doctors themselves, it was unsound. Peace of mind is important in the treatment of TB – as it is in the treatment of any illness – but especially so for tuberculosis, because prolonged convalescence implies prolonged and therefore more debilitating anxiety. The question then is why Moore and his colleagues did not a) negotiate some arrangements for the welfare of the dependents of evacuees, and b) ensure good communications between southern patients and northern kin by assigning this job to someone – especially during the years before the policy of concentration, when individuals were scattered among many hospitals.

There is, in the written record, much urging of this problem upon their superiors by the EAP doctors themselves. But of the discussion that must have gone on over their heads, there does not appear to be any report. The reliability and most of all the fullness of the textual record is never sure. Many circumstances may be omitted; nor is it possible to gauge how much pressure from the judgements of anticipated future readers, as opposed to immediate ones, each rapporteur felt when sitting down to write.

As for the Inuit view of the events, it seems not to have been recorded at the time. Now, however, it is possible that information is to be found among the recollections gathered in the course of various projects to preserve the experience of elders. So accounts have likely been collected but not yet systematically examined.[127]

If it is the case that a joint history of events (even in the form of an explicit agreement to disagree) is necessary for reconciliation (once more, always assuming it is needed or desired) then we are still at a distance from such an understanding of the evacuations. It has been difficult to learn why the senior doctors at Health and Welfare did not plan for the consequences of sudden evacuation. Attributing bad behaviour to a putative colonialist mentality explains nothing, is circular and, in this case, would be contradictory, since medical paternalism implies care, not disregard. Perhaps there was reliance on the old triad of the company, the missions and the Mounties, especially the last, to deal with the disruptions. Perhaps financial considerations were important. Then too, the attitudes of Moore and his closer collaborators should enter the account. Moore seems to have been temperamentally inclined to the technical solution, and was necessarily, as an administrator laying long-term plans and a veteran of the Great Depression, very sensitive to costs. But there is little biographical information on these men, who were few in number and therefore unusually influential in determining what was attempted.

4.

It was recognized early on that the *Howe* was inadequate as a medical vehicle, and arrangements were made to supplement the survey, examination and vaccination work with other ships and planes. In the mid-sixties planes were used for rapid evacuation of patients first gathered on the ship, and served repatriation as well. The summary medical report for the 1958 EAP begins by noting that two adults and nine children scheduled for repatriation from Hamilton were sent straight to Frobisher Bay by air. The price was $1,422, as opposed to the $1,408 it would have cost to carry them on the *Howe* – exclusive of nursery care of the children. In 1959, for the first time, more people were repatriated than were brought out (five hundred ninety-nine versus five hundred twenty-four). More importantly, of three hundred twenty evacuated from the Eastern Arctic, two hundred fifty were sent by field staff, working through the year, rather than by the doctors of the itinerant EAP team[128] – despite the fact that the patrol was becoming more and more a medical venture, and the *Howe* had few supply obligations between Montreal and Churchill. Much travel was by air. Twenty-one were put off at Port Harrison to be flown to Moose Factory General Hospital. Thirteen were to be flown by the RCAF from Resolute to Hamilton, but bad weather forced them to Clearwater instead. Twenty more were to fly out of Frobisher Bay while forty went on the *Howe*. And the brusqueness had been moderated: "two patients were left at Clyde River for subsequent evacuation due to inabilities of the welfare personnel to arrange adequate foster parentage for involved children. This inability in no way reflects upon the professional zeal of the welfare worker, but is attributable totally to inadequate working time."[129]

Other changes were unfolding. The medical officer on the *Howe* in that year also doubled as the senior administrative officer. Northern Affairs supplied a junior officer, as well as an interpreter and a medical social worker. Coordination was finally achieved – at least on paper. The urgency of the TB campaign was fading, the methods changing – a little too rapidly for Moore. On receiving the report of the 1963 patrol, he learned that a "reactivated case of tuberculosis refused evacuation and was left at Broughton Island with a year's supply of INH and PAS." Moore did not like it, feeling that Broughton Island was too isolated for this approach. Indeed, the whole trend made him uneasy:

> Dr. Shepherd mentions that Dr. Robertson tended to place "a considerable number" of patients on outpatient therapy and that one year's supply of drugs was given to each such patient. Reports on outpatient therapy even among the more sophisticated groups suggest that many cease to take the drugs within the first three months and it is suggested that in isolated areas, it might be safer to bring south for treatment any patient for whom it is considered necessary to prescribe a year's course of treatment. Perhaps you would like to discuss this matter with Dr. Wherett.[130]

The relaxed attitude that troubled Moore was a long way from the uncertainties of the forties, when the scope of the TB problem was not even known, and still further from the high anxiety of the Willis-Phillips patrol of 1955, when evacuation was so strongly urged, and treatment was mainly streptomycin by injection, along with one or two unpleasant companion drugs.

The shift toward exclusive medical use of the *Howe* continued until 1965 when the ship was dedicated solely to health and welfare concerns. No cargo was carried for the Montreal–Churchill stretch, and the use of the ship as a temporary hotel for stevedores was stopped.[131] That same year, a long-standing practice in the Western Arctic, the spring medical survey by air, came East. It was conducted in April by Norman Harper from a Douglas DC-3 chartered from Nordair.

Harper started at Frobisher Bay on April 13, collecting film and equipment. On April 14, the plane took him to Hall Beach. With him were a doctor and an Inuit darkroom technician. They were met by two nurses and an RCAF man who ferried them about on a snowmobile. The local RCMP officer served as registrar, and one hundred sixteen were x-rayed. The next day it was on to Igloolik, to screen another one hundred twenty-two. The following day the party visited camps in the area, where much smaller numbers were seen – twenty-one at one place, eight in another and twelve in a third. The snowmobile had been transported with them in the plane. "This was a very good idea," Harper thought, "as the plane could not land too close to some of the camps. As we were setting up in the plane, Const. Donahue and an interpreter would go to the camp and collect the people, usually returning towing a sled behind the skidoo."[132]

The same procedure was followed for other regions around Baffin centred on Clyde River and Lake Harbour. On April 27, the survey returned to Frobisher Bay and x-rayed the students at a couple of schools. In total, Harper had x-rayed a thousand people, including thirty-six whites in thirteen locations over twelve days. That summer, the *Howe* took nine weeks to do 3,100. (The *Howe*'s dentists were very busy, performing 478 restorations and 862 extractions after examining

2,920 patients – an ominous indication of a transition in diet and general health.[133])

By August 1968 the facts were these: "The annual costs [of EAP] to the department is estimated at $42,000 and we can carry out two air surveys of the area at a lesser cost and with the high incidence of Tuberculosis in the Eastern Arctic, two surveys a year are considered necessary: 57 new and 19 relapsed cases were discovered in Baffin Zone in 1967 and . . . there were 83 patients hospitalized (Weston 53, Moose Factory 30)."[134]

Three successful Easter air surveys had been carried out. Dentists and ophthalmologists went in once a year by air. The cost of regular bimonthly visits to major settlements by a doctor was $54,000, money that was lacking. Accordingly, it was suggested that the 1968 patrol be the *Howe*'s last, and that reliance be placed in aircraft instead, with a second annual survey to be done by Twin Otter planes on floats in the autumn.

The end of the patrol inaugurated in 1922 was announced to the larger medical community in the *Canadian Medical Association Journal* [*CMAJ*] for March 1969, in tones of some regret:

> Three generations of Canadian physicians have participated in this annual event which combined their professional skills with a spirit of high adventure . . .
>
> The decision to halt the annual Eastern Arctic Medical Patrol ends a tradition and opens a new era in the North. (Hicks, 537–38)

However, "the North Star still beckon[ed]" (ibid., 538), for seven ships continued to operate in those fabled waters, and each needed a doctor.

FOUR: THE CAPTIVITY

1.

Although set apart as a place of rest and quiet, the Mountain Sanatorium was a very busy place indeed in the early days of combination chemotherapy. Eighteen months of accelerating turnover was followed by an influx of a completely new kind of patient. The air- and sealift brought Inuit to and from the North, and nurses streamed in from Europe, joined by doctors and other specialists who were visiting or recruited as permanent staff by the superintendent on trips abroad. The place was a crossroads and cultural bazaar for northerners, southerners and so-called new Canadians alike. The Inuit encountered television and lipstick, and their caregivers encountered the Inuit and enjoyed an atmosphere of egalitarianism and collegiality still fondly recalled for interviewers. Some of these women were as well-travelled as their patients.

Nurse Gerda Van Wanrooy journeyed with her family from Holland to Picture Butte, AB, and thence, after a stint in the sugar beet fields where they relieved Japanese internees now freed from wartime bondage, to Hamilton and the San. (Preceded here also by the Japanese, of whom twenty-five had been set to work as orderlies, cleaners, kitchen staff and laundry helpers to ease wartime labour shortages.[135]) Johanna van der Woerd, also Dutch, began her Canadian career in Hamilton, went on to Moose Factory hospital for two years and then returned to Mountain Sanatorium, later to do a tour with the EAP on the *Howe*. Hilda Ferrier, who had nursed in London through the war, afterward went to Poole Sanatorium in Middlesborough, UK, before coming to Hamilton in 1952. Kathe Neuman, a physiotherapist trained in Munich, was recruited in 1954, and made return trips to Germany to recruit others once established as head of physiotherapy here.

Similarly many of the doctors came from afar, stayed for a year or two and then moved on. After studies at Budapest and Leipzig, Germany, Ferenc Bender received his medical diploma in 1937, and a diploma in public health in 1939. Familiar with TB work, he was sent to Germany in 1942, where he was senior resident at a hospital attached to the University of Berlin. In 1949 he came to Canada and qualified to practise here the following year. He then went to the Royal Edward Laurentian Hospital in Sainte-Agathe-des-Monts, QC, before returning to Hamilton. Tak Cheung graduated from Lingnan University in Canton, China, and came to Canada in 1948, where he received a diploma in public health at the University of Toronto. He joined the staff of Mountain Sanatorium for six months, then went to England, before returning to Canada to work at the Brant Sanatorium in Brantford, ON. Menna Lemoine was at Mountain San for five years, following stints at sanatoria in Corner Brook, NL; Lethbridge, AB; and Wilson, NC – but she started in TB work with an eighteen-month tour at the Camsell, in the winter of 1949/50.[136]

Unlike the Inuit, however, the immigrants had chosen change, and continued past that choice within a stable background of expectations. (Excepting, of course, the fluctuations of TB treatment itself, in which it was not easy, after 1953 or so, to plan a career.) They could even return, if they wished, to their homeland and revisit their choice. The Inuit could not return at a time of their own choosing, and when they did go back, much had changed and even the stable background of nature, the land and the animals, might be less accessible to them than before. Their sojourn, for better or worse, was a captivity.

Mountain Sanatorium was a village of one thousand four hundred or so souls – half of them patients, of all ages, and half of these Inuit – presided over by Hugo and Ellen Ewart, a brother and sister team who were medical superintendent and head of nursing, respectively, assisted by Ernest Bell, the business manager. The institution was sustained over the years by ever-growing endowments; the continuous gifts of a host of volunteers, organized and not; and the long-standing involvement of the local notables. Havoc had been wrought upon the organization by streptomycin and other chemotherapy. Having secured the custom of the Indian Health Services to tide them over, however, Ewart must have sometimes felt like the proverbial dog that finally catches the car: what immediately ensues is not at all as the dog imagined.

San staff understood the challenge posed by the arrival of Inuit in large numbers, and adapted, but soon were overwhelmed because the sanatorium culture was weakened on two fronts. First, antibiotics made the rest treatment redundant, and discipline difficult to maintain; and second, cultural difference collapsed the rehabilitation programs that had become an essential adjunct of the rest treatment. As for the Inuit, along with many other new things and persons, they also met themselves. Nelson Graburn, the anthropologist and lifelong student of Inuit expression, puts it succinctly. During the period of several generations when the northerners knew of the Europeans and adopted some of their products, change was slow:

> Nevertheless, the very knowledge of another way of life and the cultural changes undertaken introduced a heightened self-consciousness among Inuit about their own culture . . . The very self-consciousness about difference may have worked to erode some aspects of Inuit traditional culture . . .
>
> . . . [Of course] "culture" is far from being constituted by an array of traits that can be selected or "saved" at will . . .
>
> Awareness of the erosion of Inuit traditional culture and language arose across the North in many ways and was experienced differently in different ones and even by particular individuals. Those Inuit who were taken south for tuberculosis treatment or for education or other reasons often got to know white people "as people" and to visit their homes and see their families. From the 1950s on their tales were spread far and wide . . .

This intimacy and the "education" of those who had lived "down south" brought up the possibility of speaking English not just as a limited-purpose trade language but as a true alternative . . . One result was a conscious movement to preserve the language though various political actions in the Eastern Arctic, including having the first years of schooling conducted in Inuttitut [*sic*]. Eventually some adults, even if bilingual, consciously started speaking Inuttitut to children all the time. (Graburn, 140–41)

It is widely asserted that the southern interlude marked an epoch in the history of Nunavut and Nunavik, but it is not so easy to determine just what occurred. No patient records are held at Hamilton Health Sciences, the successor to the Hamilton Health Association that ran the San. Discharge sheets were kept, but these are still treated as active medical records and are inaccessible. Sample records were kept at Weston, and one will be drawn on in a later section of this chapter. There seems to have been no study of the episode undertaken at the time, although there was recognition that this was a special situation, in which the people were uniquely available to outsiders – in some respects an anthropologist's or linguist's paradise, in fact. This is what it seems to have been for Raymond Gagné, recruited to the education department in September 1954, who began working on his M.A. thesis in linguistics. However, the concern was more for what could be taught than what could be learned; Euro-Canadian authority then, and for another decade after, regarded Aboriginal Canadians mainly as potential dependents requiring supervision in hospital and out, rather than essential partners – as they had been in the past. There were exceptions. In the spring of 1958 Frank Vallee, then an assistant professor of sociology at McMaster, proposed to enter this "little world on its own" as a participant observer in the employ of Northern Affairs, lightly disguised as a teacher of English. Vallee requested funding to spend six months looking at the effect of hospital life on the patients.

To the majority of people in our society who are hospitalized there are clear-cut and well known understandings about why they are there, about how they should behave and be treated . . . At the end of their confinement in hospital, they move back into a world in which, after suitable convalescence, most of them have a meaningful, familiar role to play. What about the patient whose pre- and post-hospital way of life is highly discontinuous with that of the hospital? What are the short-term and long-term effects of lengthy hospitalization on such persons? What can be done to render the effects of hospitalization less disruptive? What can be done to take fullest advantage of the "captive" situation to engender desirable social and psychological changes?[137]

Equally valuable would have been Vallee's proposed second stage, field work "devoted to studying some long-term effects of hospitalization in people who have been patients but have returned to the North."[138] Nothing seems to have come of this, though Vallee went on to co-edit a collection of Arctic Studies, *Eskimo of the Canadian Arctic*, and worked extensively in the North.

Another anthropologist alert to the possibilities offered by the evacuation and concentration policy was Svend Frederiksen, a Greenlander and fluent Inuktitut speaker whose interest was in the body of knowledge held by shamans. In August 1957 Frederiksen visited Mountain San to converse with elderly Inuit patients. Subsequently Frederiksen sought informants both in northern villages and in southern sanatoria, visiting the sanatorium in Ninette, MB; the Clearwater Lake Sanatorium in The Pas, and perhaps also the Charles Camsell as he passed through Edmonton on his way to Alaska in the summer of 1959 (d'Anglure, Hansen and Frederiksen).[139]

By 1962 it was all over in Hamilton. The Mountain San had shrunk to a single building – the others had been adapted to new uses. There was or would be a chronic care centre, a children's hospital, a large and up-to-the-minute laboratory, a technical school, a nursing school and a rehabilitation centre. The care of Inuit TB patients was passed over to the Weston Sanatorium in Toronto, and the Ontario minister of health convened a special two-day meeting of sanatoria superintendents and other public health administrators to talk about the "division in the road" at which they found themselves – that is, coping with "a trend to less hospitalization, less sanatorium care and more treatment in the home or in the community setting with anti-tuberculosis drugs, resulting in a problem as to the successful application of those drugs and this form of therapy."[140]

2.

When Johanna van der Woerd came to Canada in 1954, her first nursing job was at Nora-Frances Henderson Hospital in Hamilton. She hated it. People were so harsh and rude that she was stung to tears. Moreover, although she was already a fully qualified and duly registered nurse, she was employed as a lowly nursing assistant and treated as a lesser being. She left and went to Mountain Sanatorium, which was another world (personal interview).

Here there were no lesser beings, and everyone was made to feel at home. All agree that the absence of social distance at the San was remarkable and much appreciated by everyone lucky enough to experience it. In the dining room the nurses, doctors, cleaning staff and technicians all sat together. Ellen Ewart, head of nursing, lived in one of the nurses' residences along with the women she supervised. Along with her brother, Hugo, the medical super, and Ernest Bell, the business manager, Ewart was the public face of a stable cadre who remained in place throughout the turmoil of the fifties. In 1955, at the fullest extent of its expansion, the institution spread over three hundred seventy acres. Excluding the farm buildings, but including the powerhouse, kitchen and laundry, the San counted fifteen buildings in two clusters – one, of five, at the brow of the escarpment; the remainder grouped nearly a kilometre to the south. The newest was the Holbrook Pavilion, opened at the end of 1951. It housed the San's school, and had sixty beds for children and a nurse's residence on a second floor. The oldest buildings were the Brow Infirmary, opened in 1916, and two nearby pavilions built in 1917 for returned soldiers. The largest was the Evel building, with one hundred eighty-five beds.

Medical records, radiology, bronchoscopy, dentistry and the canteen were on the ground floor. The third and fourth floors were operating and recovery rooms. Adjacent was the Southam Pavilion, whose basement housed the laboratory and the morgue.

Ewart, the spokesman and ubiquitous flag carrier, was continuously reaching out. In addition to recruiting and hiring, he seems to have attended every internal event or function, every social tea or entertainment, every retirement party or christening, and was out and about in town as well. While Ewart raised funds and maintained the San's presence in the minds of Hamiltonians great and small, and Bell and a small staff spent the money and kept the accounts, the medical work was done principally by the trio of David Aitchison, Paul Rabinowitz and Arthur Armstrong, supported by a large nursing staff. Backing up the lab was the pharmacy, overseen by Grace Macdonald. Other medical people were also present over the long term, notably Doctors Lee and H. E. Peart (and at the very end Reginald Empey), but the trend was toward shorter stints. By the early sixties, a number of separate institutions had inherited the functions and the buildings that the San had aggregated during its fifty-year span. A children's hospital was launched, and a rehabilitation centre, and a school of radiology and medical technology.

At the apogee, however, in the mid-fifties, with over seven hundred patients in residence, the scale of operations was grand. In 1953, twenty-two thousand x-ray films were made in the course of ten thousand investigations – seven hundred of these were for bone and joint troubles. Meanwhile the lab processed sixty-five thousand tests and analyses, of which about twenty-seven thousand were bacteriological.[141] Figures are difficult to find for chemotherapy, but since streptomycin, PAS and INH were in use, the number of doses given would have been in the hundreds every day, with strep injections continuing twice a week for at least a year for each patient. The preparation and administration of these substances was carried through by the nursing staff under the direction of Ellen Ewart, who arrived in 1938 as assistant superintendent, became head of nursing in 1939 and stayed for twenty-three years. Her brother, who was in his job until 1970, came to the San in 1945 as an assistant to the medical superintendent, Dr. Brig. Cecil H. Playfair, with whom he had worked in England during World War II. Ewart maintained a private practice until Playfair died unexpectedly two years later, and his assistant was quickly appointed in his place. Ewart had started out in economics and history and worked in efficiency studies for the Goodyear and Firestone tire companies before going into medicine. At one time or another he was on the board of the Hamilton-Wentworth Children's Aid Society, the Canadian Cancer Society, the Humane Society, the Hamilton Chamber of Commerce and the Rotary Club of Hamilton. He also served as president of the Ontario Medical Association and the Ontario Tuberculosis Association. This list is incomplete. Keeping track of extra-medical matters was Ernest Bell, who, from 1951 on, reported to Ewart on accounting, purchasing and stores, diet, housekeeping, roads and engineering, the garage, the farm, the canteen, the mail service, and buildings and grounds. Just to be sure that nothing got past him, he was also made secretary of the San's school board, which had about twenty people on the payroll in 1954.[142]

Head of medicine was Joseph Lee, who fell ill while with the EAP on the *Howe* in 1959, and had to be airlifted out, dying shortly after. Surgery was Aitchison, backed by George Yang. Aitchison had been a Canadian pilot in the Royal Air Force in 1918. After the war he studied medicine in Toronto, London and Berlin. Back home in 1927 he contracted TB and was out of action for three years, had a pneumothorax and a phrenic crush, and signed on at Mountain Sanatorium in 1931, where he continued until 1964 when his TB flared up again. While he was off dealing with it, his replacement was H. J. Sullivan, yet another TB doctor with first-hand experience of the disease. Stricken while in med school, Sullivan had a pneumothorax and kept going for refills to maintain one lung in a collapsed state for five years straight. This was just the beginning of his career as a patient, which went on intermittently for a good ten years. He left surgery at the San in 1952, but carried on with chest work in the city.

His replacement was Yang, who actually displaced Aitchison as chief operator. Between 1952 and 1960 he performed 1,978 operations at the San, of which four hundred eighty-eight were thoracic surgeries (Delarue, 165). That is, Yang carried out one major chest operation every week for eight years, which is rather amazing. Yang, born in 1914, was about fifteen years younger than Aitchison. His medical school was Cheeloo University in Shandong, a coastal province of China. After serving four years with an ambulance unit he came to Canada in 1948 and became assistant surgeon at the San in 1952. Antibiotics changed the character of surgery, as smaller lesions meant smaller resections. Aitchison and Yang specialized in resection with concomitant thoracoplasty, that is, the concurrent removal of lung tissue and ribs, which collapsed the operated-on lung and allowed it to rest. This double procedure reduced post-operative problems (Delarue, 160–67).

As there are no accessible records, it is impossible at present to know the extent of surgical treatment among evacuees. This is unfortunate, as it would allow us to better determine how many of the evacuees absolutely needed to be in southern Canada, owing to the demands of surgery and recovery. Some pulmonary cases would have had major operations, but the only available reference is anecdotal. Joe Stark, a lung cancer patient, was admitted in 1957. While awaiting surgery, he drew strength from the example, as he told Aitchison, of a young Inuk he had met. "You've taken out her right lung and you've taken out one lobe from her left lung. She's got one lobe and she's running around here like a little blue housefly" (quoted in Ralph Holland Wilson, 185).

Supporting the surgeons were the bronchoscopist and the laboratory technicians. The first was Paul Rabinowitz, the ear, nose and throat specialist. Of Russian origins, Rabinowitz studied in Berlin and came to Canada in 1926. In 1928 he joined the staff at the San and remained for the rest of his career, with interruptions during World War II and again in 1949 when he went to Holland for four months of in-hospital study, stopping in England for a couple of weeks on his way home.[143] Heading the lab was Riley A. Armstrong, whose staff of twenty not only performed an enormous quantity of tests and analyses, but assisted in research as well, conducting two studies on

PAS and resistance, and another on INH acetylation rates. Building on the work of his predecessor, W. Stuart Stanbury (a blood bank expert), Armstrong developed a huge museum collection of specimens and slides. At an international conference held in Toronto in 1961, the lab presented an exhibit of two hundred fifty-nine slides detailing their procedures and the pathology of the disease: dyeing and identification of the bacillus, cultivation of TB and other mycobacterium, testing for drug resistance, specimen collection and samples of a variety of lesions. Armstrong also developed a method of embedding body cross-sections in plastic, and the resulting collection passed to the medical school (Delarue, 161).

3.

The sanatorium program on the eve of the Inuit arrival was first of all segregation and regimentation – so-called sanatorium routine. This might have been supplemented with collapse therapy or surgical intervention to remove hopelessly damaged tissues, or to repair hips or spines. Segregation was enforced even within the San itself, with infants and young children being separated from their mothers and placed in another ward or even with foster parents in the community.

The average stay around 1950 was fifteen months (four hundred sixty-one days). Mild disease might be cleared up in eleven months.[144] The length of stay was actually increasing, probably due to the early effects of the antibiotics on the disease pool, as they saved or prolonged the lives of hard-hit patients previously doomed. In 1950 over half of the dead or discharged received streptomycin with PAS, made free to all thanks to a federal grant provided from 1948 on (Brink, 25). By 1952 seventy-five percent of all patients discharged had received streptomycin (Wicks, "Recent Trends in Treatment and in Operating Funds at Tuberculosis Hospitals in Ontario"). However, "bed rest in a recumbent position with graded exercise categories ordered by the attending physicians" remained the basic treatment (Wicks, "Sanatorium Treatment of Tuberculosis Patients in Ontario"), and was still cherished by staff at the Weston Sanatorium in the early sixties, when incoming Inuit were advised in English and syllabics that

> tuberculosis heals by "scarring," that is replacement of the diseased area by scar tissue. You have probably seen this scarring when you had a cut. Pulling or stretching of the healing area will keep breaking or tearing this scar . . . Rest to the part affected is the best method of healing . . . In tuberculosis of the lungs you cannot put the lungs completely to rest . . . But by lying quietly in bed we can make the size of the lungs smaller and stretch it as little as possible.[145]

The exercise grades ranged from Total Bed Grade Zero – "no sitting up, self-care to be done in recumbent position, reading, listening to radio or light occupational therapy only in recumbent position" – to Grade Three – "may sit up in bed for one hour, in two periods, daily" – and on through "bathroom once, twice, or three times daily"; "full bathroom"; "church" and finally, after several more steps, the ultimate "evening privileges." This last entitled one to stay up until nine.[146]

A patient chart from Weston Sanatorium, showing the frequency and dosage of medications, and variations in temperature. Courtesy of the Godfrey L. Gale Archives and Museum, West Park Healthcare Centre, Toronto.

The rationale for extreme rest followed from autopsy observations that cavities and dead tissue occurred mainly in the upper third of the lung.

> It was postulated that three mechanical factors prevented healing of such cavities: the surrounding lung's static elastic recoil maintaining traction at the cavity's walls and thus preventing collapse, dynamically increased traction from breathing, and upright posture leading to preferentially decreased apical blood and lymph flow. Bed rest worked on three fronts: it reduced functional residual capacity and thus static tension; it decreased ventilation and thus dynamic traction; and it improved apical perfusion by eliminating the pressure gradient promoted by upright posture . . . exercise was like arsenic: valuable in small defined doses for certain patients under a doctor's close supervision but dangerously fatal to anyone else. (McCuaig, 69)[147]

If rest was imperative then best of all would be to render the diseased lung inactive altogether, and this was the result sought through the collapse therapies, chiefly induced pneumothorax, which involved aspirating by vacuum bottle from around the lung, and simultaneously allowing air or some other fluid to enter and occupy the same space. The effect was to collapse the lung and free it from the motions of breathing. In the event that an adhesion prevented collapse, a secondary operation was performed to cut the tie. This was pneumolysis. The pneumothorax procedure was spontaneously reversible, so refills were needed at intervals to keep the lung flattened. Not so with thoracoplasty, the next turn of the screw, where ribs were removed to release all of the support to which tissue could adhere and so hold open a cavity. With the anchor gone, the lung tissue shifted and the hole closed up and hopefully healed.

Variations on these two operations were more or less drastic. Pneumothorax was popular during the thirties but tapered away after 1945. Thoracoplasty, meanwhile, doubled in application in Ontario between 1946 and 1950, peaking in that year when about fifteen percent of all persons discharged from TB hospitals alive had undergone the procedure (Wicks, "Sanatorium Treatment of Tuberculosis Patients in Ontario.").[148] Finally, collapse therapy was potentially made redundant by a technique crossing over from a parallel train of development. This happened around 1945 when Alvan L. Barach had the idea that a machine designed to assist respiration could also be useful in unloading the lungs of TB patients. The machine in question was the barospirator, invented in 1926 by Torsten Thunberg in Lund, Sweden. By enclosing his patient in an airtight chamber and then varying the pressure, Thunberg could churn gases without having to call upon the chest to do much work. Barach wanted no work at all, so he made some changes and produced the equalizing alternating pressure chamber or lung immobilizer.

"When patients have learned to dispense with voluntary breathing," Barach explained, "the impulse for spontaneous muscular movement is remarkably diminished; in some cases no movement of the arms or legs is observed for hours at a time . . . boredom is not complained of and . . . patients are for the most part willing to carry on the treatment without entertainment." This continued for ten hours a day, in varying blocks of time, for four months or more. Clearly this was not going to be cheap, or widely applicable, but the experimenters had had very good results with persons whose lung cavities were not shrinking under any other treatment. These were gaping holes four centimetres across, which, owing to prolonged rest of the lung, were made to disappear when all else had failed, and without any need for surgery and its risks (Cullen et al.). Never laggard, the Hamilton Health Association stepped up, and the *Hamilton Spectator* for January 19, 1950, ran a photo of the San's Dr. Ian Harper contemplating the newly acquired Emerson lung immobilizer, one of only two in the country. It was a beauty, sleek and cylindrical, with a Plexiglas viewport and head section – and even then almost obsolete, marginalized by the ascendant wonder drugs.

The importance of rest, however, persisted in the minds of doctors through the 1960s. Julius H. Comroe, Jr., wrote a history column called Retrospectroscope for *The American Review of Respiratory Disease*. In one of these articles he set out the twists and turns of TB treatment by reviewing medical textbooks from about 1890 until 1975. The standard *Cecil-Loeb Textbook of Medicine* was still big on bedrest in 1955, after strep, PAS and INH had come into wide use. By 1959 chemo had seven pages of discussion but bedrest was still highly recommended as an accompaniment. Not until 1963 did *Cecil-Loeb* allow that, with the right drugs, the further effect of rest was negligible (Comroe).

Rest was to be mental as well as physical, so good care meant the provision of amenities that would keep up morale. These included good mail service, regular movies and concerts, the earphone system for delivery of radio directly to each bed, a library, a patients' council, a patient newsletter and beautification of the grounds. It also meant the maintenance of a program of educational and occupational therapy – rehabilitation services, in short, to reassure the patient that they had a life beyond the San.

Once the Inuit had been placed in controlled surroundings under tight discipline, the problems of rehabilitation with a view to repatriation came to the fore. At first, there was confidence in the very well established and thoroughgoing services already present – and in fact they were so good that Ewart credited them with swinging the decision to concentrate Inuit in Hamilton.

Occupational therapy (OT) had been introduced by the Department of Soldiers' Civil Re-Establishment during the First World War, partly to help maintain discipline among the returned soldiers who made for restless and sometimes defiant patients. By 1919 ten therapists – plus teachers in motor mechanics, woodworking, drafting and music – were working with one hundred fifty patients. But these activities hovered between vocational training and mere busy work. Subsequently, the regular school curriculum was made available and steadily expanded so that in the academic year of 1952/53, patients were able to acquire even university credits, though the bulk of the courses were still in technical subjects such as typing and shorthand, blueprint reading and machine drawing, radio and electricity. Education, even without the promise of employment, was more dignified than say basket weaving, but took time – the prescribed coursework had to be completed and so the program of study was of a necessary minimum duration. However, leather craft and carving afforded the dignity of employment, and so participation, because the product was saleable. The craftsman enjoyed recognition and tangible benefits – cash toward the purchase of canteen goods – which soothed the nagging ache of dependence.

In mid-1956, the rehabilitation program was divided into OT and physiotherapy; the former attached to the education department, while physio was paired with surgery. (Post-operative physiotherapy was needed for hip, spine and lung cases. Patients of the latter, during recovery from thoracoplasty, had to be taught how to offset their body's tendency to reshape itself around the missing ribs. Otherwise the shoulder on the operated side would rise and come forward.)

However, to the extent that OT meant some sort of job training or academic qualification, it was problematic for many Inuit. Very few had completed or even begun primary education, and it was unclear for what they should train. Some radio and watch repair was taught out west, but those patients had to stay on in southern Canada when cured in order to find work. Ironically, carving, rather a useless skill when compared to say, small engine repair, turned out the most successful means of producing a commodity. The women's sewing was more obviously valuable. Along with dolls and appliqué work on decorative hangings, which were offered for sale locally alongside the men's carvings, they made duffle parkas for returnees – everyone got new clothing on discharge – and pyjamas for the institution, being paid by the piece. They were taught the Euro-Canadian practice of sewing to measured patterns, using a graduated tape rather than a length of string, which was the Inuit usage. There was also a season of parachute sewing.[149] Similarly, in 1958, in conjunction with efforts to establish the commercial char fishery at George River (now Kangiqsualujjuaq, QC); Port Burwell (now Killiniq, NT) and Frobisher Bay (now Iqaluit, NU), net making was introduced for the men.

Fine art carving and rehab carving were intertwined from the outset, but two parallel and different systems of retailing the product developed, and by the mid-fifties the hospital product was becoming a threat to quality control in the more tightly managed and prosperous art world. But artistic production was helpful to sanatoria-bound Inuit.

Staffed entirely by volunteers and managed gratis by its founder, Thelma Poag, the sanatorium shop in 1955 was doing $8,200 a year in doll's clothing, jewellery, soapstone carving, stuffed toys (cranked out by a four-woman team), leather goods and other items (Waller).[150] The San advanced materials and tools, and reclaimed that amount from eventual sales. The shop took five percent. Earnings were paltry but still meaningful for patients given the canteen prices: seven cents for a coke, a dollar for a flashlight, fifteen cents for batteries, twenty-five dollars for a radio. Lipstick was seventy cents, cameras ten to fifteen dollars, film fifty cents. Snackers could pick up a tin of corn beef for fifty cents or a can of peaches for twenty-two.[151]

But the question of quality was urgent if carving was to bring in real, steady money, and life beyond the hospital was not cheap. Around 1960 a barrel of fuel oil at Cape Dorset went for twenty-eight dollars, more at remoter places. At Coral Harbour (Salliq in Inuktitut) a twenty-two-foot canoe was $625, and a 7.5-horsepower outboard motor was $275. A Peterhead boat would set you back $10,000 (Jenness). The average price for a fox pelt over the decade in the entire territory was about thirteen dollars. According to HBC man Duncan Pryde, his post was paying about twenty dollars a pelt and this was also the cost of a good untrained pup. A trapper needed a team of fifteen or more dogs (Pryde, 158). If art was going to account for anything in the North, it would have to command fine art prices.

Here and there in the literature one comes upon references to the great mechanical aptitude of the Inuit. According to Edmund Carpenter, writing in 1973, it was in fact seriously under-reported.

> If arctic literature rarely mentions the Eskimo's mechanical aptitude, it is simply because it is so often silent about those things which are taken for granted about Eskimo life. Yet all observers to whom I have spoken agree there is something here not easily explained. I have heard many stories about Eskimo mechanics, some difficult to credit were it not for the fact that such achievements can be observed daily.

Aivilik men are first-class mechanics. They delight in stripping down and reassembling engines, watches, all machinery . . . No engine is beyond repair.

If one man starts working on an engine, the men and boys of the camp crowd close about, talking and helping. Once they see how to fix it, they rarely forget. I think the first thing that impresses them about Western culture is its machinery. (30–31)

In a memoir, Minnie Aodla Freeman mentioned an incident involving her brother. One evening he was very late returning from the family's nets. The next day he told his sister privately that having dropped the outboard motor in the water, he had to take it entirely apart, dry each piece and reassemble it. She was amazed he could do it, and he said he had learned by watching his father and memorizing his moves.

This way of learning, by observation and exact repetition, common to farm children and apprentices in Euro-Canadian society, is in contrast to the methods of trial and error, and progressive approximation generally used in formal schooling. However, some knowledge is not learnable by observation, because the opportunity to do so does not exist; that is, some knowledge is not readily modelled. Not that the northerners were complete strangers to book learning; far from it. The literacy rate was high – ninety percent – and bible reading was widespread. But some took to the academic style better than others – Mary Panigusiq and Minnie Aodla Freeman, for example. However, there were also elements of Inuit intellectual culture that were portable, and lay between the machine and the book. String games and bone games were about figuration and naming, and offered training in observation. There were a great many named string figures, of differing complexity and difficulty. Bone games, using seal flipper bones were played by laying out the bones to form a pattern – either the articulation they had in life, or glyphs: dog, man, lamp and so on. It seems odd that neither string nor bone games appear in any photographs of San life. These pastimes, exercises in memory and dexterity that allowed parents to know the inward character and capacities of their children, would have been helpful also in sustaining the language skills of the younger patients.

4.

The Inuit were preceded, in October 1954, by a contingent of fifty-one Cree from Moose Factory General Hospital, overcrowded as it was and functioning both as a general and a TB hospital.[152] In December the advance guard of Inuit, twenty-four strong, arrived by train. They were transferees from Parc Savard, escorted by Dr. J. E. Labrecque himself, bearing with him the relevant x-ray photos. Anglican Archdeacon R. C. Blagrave was on hand to greet them. Presumably these patients were already accustomed to sanatorium discipline. The next bunch, Ewart told the *Hamilton Spectator*, would be coming "right out of the igloo."[153]

The prospect was at first exciting for education department staff, who like everyone else faced unemployment if patient numbers fell too far. But when the wild ones began arriving – by November of 1955 there were three hundred thirty-five Inuit in residence – the reality was disappointing. Not for the nurses, who found the newcomers obliging, cheerful and affectionate; nor for the clergy, who had a captive congregation, mostly Anglican. But the encounter with a mass of mostly unschooled country people of all ages, pretty well devoid of English, overwhelmed the educators. The brevity of the stays made rehab by education less and less relevant overall, especially for the locals. Nevertheless in 1962 the remaining few Inuit patients were taking thirty-nine subjects to complement the informal and involuntary education they were receiving in dress and comportment from their small-town Euro-Canadian surroundings, from magazines and from television – an appliance not yet available in the North.

What stands out in the San program is a shift in attitudes toward Aboriginal languages and to what is now called cultural persistence. Aboriginals enter the San's written records for the first time in their own voices in August 1955, with four greetings that appeared in the mimeographed patient newsletter, *Mountain Views*. A page of handwritten Cree syllabics was followed by a page of English translation, and began, "I am Lily Pepabano. I come from Fort George, Quebec." Next, "I am Lottie Spence. I come from Attawapiskat, James Bay."[154]

Over the page there is more, but these writers are Inuit: Tom Talouk and Leah Palliser. "At the beginning of October," wrote Tom (who was from Port Harrison), "we put out snares and traps for foxes." Leah wanted readers to know that "since I've come to the San, I've been on Evel 4, Evel 2, Wilcox 4, Brow 1 and now Southam 1."

The next issue (Autumn 1955) contained several more pages of Cree and Inuktitut, as well as portraits of the authors and their translators. In this way the reader met Albert Mattinas, Cree of Attawapiskat, and Kolonla, Inuit from Lake Harbour. Also Annie Koolatolik, nurse's aide from Pond Inlet, and Ann Witaltuk, an Inuit nursing student from Moose Factory. The original purpose of syllabics was also reasserted. Invented to allow converts to read the New Testament in their own tongue, the script now served to encourage the Inuit patients in the discipline of San life. Page thirty-four was a message from Miss Howting (the welfare nurse) containing a list of rules preceded by this assurance:

> Perhaps you are wondering why you are brought down from your home leaving your friends and perhaps family behind. The reason is that you are sick, and if you were left at home, you may endanger those at home. So you are here to get well again. When you are well you will go home. We are all your friends here and want to try and help you get well. Things are strange to you, our food, our hospital and even our people look different to you. But do not be afraid. Nobody here will harm you.[155]

Many familiar themes appear in these few pages. Mattinas called attention to the unhappiness of the First Nations boy in the white school. He was not free there, and did not know the food.

Another thing, this boy does not speak English so he cannot understand a thing the teacher tells him and he cannot say to the teacher why he feels puzzled and sad. I'm telling you it's very hard for him. He feels just like his father did when he was with the White Man. The White Teacher cannot understand either what is the trouble inside the young Indian boy. Nobody understands the trouble inside another person.

But the boy begins to learn that God made Indians and White Man alike to be born and to grow. He looks after us every day and wants us to pray every day.

God made Indians and White People in the same way from the same things. They feel the same way, and think the same way, all the people are all the same, not different. Everybody is all the same.

All my friends, I would like you to believe in God and to love Him.[156]

Tom Talouk, Lottie Spence and Lily Pepabano talked about hunting, as did Kolonla. They did so with a mixture of satisfaction and complaint. It was hard when the hunting was unsuccessful and it was very cold. Kolonla was concerned about his dependents: "Now here I am down here and I worry and worry about my family wondering how they are and if they're starving and who's looking after them."[157]

An editorial from Irene Howard expanded on the reasons for including this material. She explained that the syllabics pages were meant to help with the novelties of San life and to reassure distant relatives (presumably copies of the newsletter were sent northward). But there was more. Seeing the comparative easiness of Euro-Canadian life, Aboriginal people wished something similar for themselves.

But in learning our ways it is to be hoped that they will be able to retain their identity as Indian and Eskimo people. There is always a tendency for a minority people to be swallowed up in a more dominant and aggressive culture . . . certain measures have already been taken to preserve and encourage Eskimo sculpture in wood and stone and other work of Eskimo artists . . . Something should also be done to help preserve the Eskimo and Indian languages, and their traditions in song and story already dying out as the older people die and the younger generation adopt our ways. We hope our efforts in this magazine will be at least some small help in this work.[158]

Howard was expressing the confusion in white opinion that ensued when one long-standing premise was relinquished and no clear alternative was at hand. Weakened but not yet entirely absent was the naturalistic fatalism of the *vanishing American* thesis, but nothing had come to replace it except a vague folklorism. "Our ways" were still expected to prevail, but what was previously inevitable – the extinction of the old, Aboriginal ways – had become a tendency only, and against a tendency something could be done. Native languages and other artifacts could be placed before white eyes, and Aboriginals invited to speak of their own lives in their own words. Stories could be collected and recorded: Mattinas provided two, and a pair of Inuit poems were reprinted from *Canadian Eskimo Art*, a publication of the Department of Northern Affairs and Natural Resources. This exercise in multiculturalism hopefully helped in a small way by making a public display of respect for Native languages and the unique scripts in which some were written.

But if the Native was no longer vanishing, what then? Was he doubling? Or halving? Would he retain some traditions and lose others, meanwhile accumulating new ways from others? Would Inuit be "deep" Canadians, adding citizenship to the proud core of their immemorial tenure in the land? Or were they fated to be phantoms, incomplete, halflings living between two worlds and partaking fully of neither?

Four years later, in 1959, as the end of the Inuit mass sojourn in southern Canada neared, opinion was shifting again, and had become very close to current views. Under the title "Eskimos Adjust Quickly," the fitness of Inuit to modernity was emphasized by one of the San's schoolteachers in the *Bulletin of the Canadian Tuberculosis Association*.

Much print and verbal eloquence has been devoted in recent years to the explosive rapidity with which in the last two decades the traditional pattern of Eskimo life has been upset. Nobody spent much time on the fact that our ideas of the Eskimos were being jolted just as sharply, and that they were probably due for even more extensive upheaval in the next two decades. It is high time we got on with the job of absorbing the shock this will be to a generation which drew so many pictures of igloos when in grades I, II and III.

Recent visitors to the Arctic have been startled to find that there are Eskimos who prefer outboard motors to paddling their own kayaks. At Mountain Sanatorium, Hamilton, they discovered that Eskimo women adjust readily to the electric sewing machine. Ningeoapik, whose picture is on the cover, had been sewing for 60 odd years without benefit of an electric sewing machine, but she had no trouble at all getting used to it. (McKnight, "Eskimos Adjust Quickly")

Setting aside the under-informed conflation of Inuit sewing by hand on skins with the comparatively undemanding work of sewing textiles with powered machines, the keynote is the notion of "moving between cultures." The adaptability of a representative Inuk, who appeared in sensible eyewear and clenching a pipe in her teeth, was offered in evidence. Ningeoapik was credited with encouraging the children at their English lessons, as well as possessing "the most detailed and exact" knowledge of syllabics yet encountered by a teacher. Naturally the San was praised for its mediating role: "The sanatorium period has done much to help hundreds of Eskimos meet changes in their life more efficiently. If the Eskimos' readiness to accept change is sufficiently noted by fellow patients and observers it may help the rest of Canada to get adjusted to what the Arctic is to be like in the years ahead. That would also be on the credit side of the ledger" (McKnight).

This is deeply ambiguous. Inuit "readiness to accept change," their oft-reported ingenuity and adaptability, is praised here in a context in which change was not chosen but forced upon them, whether they were ready or not. But there is corroborating testimony. Here for instance is a letter to Marion McKnight, the teacher who recognized Ningeoapik's proficiency in syllabics. It was written by Joanasie Salamonie in 1996, and sent from Cape Dorset apparently in response to McKnight forwarding him some photographs.

> Dear Marion. This is real gift for me. It was so wonderful to hear from you as well as to receive photos it did bring a good memheries of youth day – when I was in Hamilton last June to attending to the memherial sevices at my father grave and many other friends whom they haved died there. And I thought of you, wondering you are still there or gone to somewhere els. Many of our friends are gone it seems that they are gone with the wind. I have wonderful family lovely grandchildren I think there [illegible] 10 grandchildren its so wonderful to have them some times. I cryed when I saw your picture it so was nice to heare from some one cared so much when I needed it in those days. I am social worker in Cape Dorset as well as alcohol counsellor. If I didn't have a good teach I know I wouldn't have made it. Again thank you. God bless Joanasie.[159]

Wanting to do good and wishing to avoid harming another is not the same as *knowing how* to do so. The recurrent, undecidable question was assimilation or not.[160] And if not, then what? The old pattern was breaking up. The tutelary determination of the would-be dominant society once again was inadequate, but this time recognition of the futility of the Euro-Canadian posture was becoming general, and caused confusion among the educators at the San.

At a meeting of the school board in January 1955, on the eve of the arrival of the first large group of evacuees, Ewart explained that

> the future of the patient was uncertain inasmuch as his physical condition might not permit him to be discharged to his home with its rigorous physical conditions and also that the decisions of the Department in Ottawa in this regard had still to be taken. The question of rehabilitation in sanatoria

centred around the basic requirements of teaching English and vocational activities of the hobby variety designed to have a therapeutic value, and second, those which might be of use in a future environment. Examples of this latter class of teaching were sewing and machine work for women, and radio and possibly the management of internal combustion engines for men . . . The Principal was then asked to outline the method by which teaching of Eskimos might be carried on. The Department had worked out a tentative scheme of operation which involved group teaching of new Canadian studies, particularly English, with elementary mathematics being introduced as soon as there was enough English to enable this to be done.[161]

By February 1957 an interpreter has been added to the occupational therapy staff, but the confident air of the early days was gone. "The question uppermost at all times is, 'What is best for the Eskimo?' Experience has led us to be very cautious."[162]

What was best for the Inuit, yes, but what was that? As Hugo Ewart recalled in 1980:

We had a big education department, I think up to 25 people, and one day the principal came over to me and said, "Look, we've got one chap – Gagné – who was a very smart chap, a lot of linguistics," and he'd come to him and said, "Look, we are doing everything wrong." We were teaching these children, a whole host of these youngsters, we were teaching them about cows and fire engines and so forth. Well what is a cow in Baffin Island? It doesn't exist and we were teaching them the usual Dick and Jane stuff.

So Raymond Gagné went to work and wrote an Eskimo primer, and he talked about little Mukluk going out to help his father seal, and so forth, and we had all this done in Eskimo. We could only send people back north at particular times of the year, so if we had a woman, an Eskimo patient who was negative [i.e., for the tuberculosis bacillus] we sent her over to the children's ward so that these children would learn Eskimo, because previously they had been going back to the north not knowing how to speak to their own parents.[163]

What Ewart remembered in 1980 is at odds with the testimony of two former child-patients, collected by Al Purdy in 1995 on the occasion of the dedication of a memorial to Inuit dead buried at Hamilton (Purdy). Both Caroline Alexander of Puvirnituq and Natsiq Alainga-Kango of Iqaluit, who arrived at the San in 1954 and 1959 respectively, reported that they lost their native tongue during their stay and had to relearn it on their return to the North. Likewise Nancy Anilniliak, recalling her time in the San during a visit to Hamilton in 2007, explained that as a six-year-old evacuee from Pangnirtung in 1959, she had learned English but forgotten her Inuktitut, except for a few words she wished to remember so as to say them to her mother on her return. Back home, she picked up her own language again quickly, and then consolidated her English at primary school.[164]

Ningeoapik, mentioned in McKnight's article, although expert in syllabics, was not keen on learning English. However, "she attended classes in which loop films were being used to teach [children] English," and exhorted the students to try harder (McKnight). Inuktitut was not mentioned, but this may be owing to the slant of the article, which was Inuit adaptability. The Gagné primer did however exist, though regrettably no copy has turned up in any archives.

Gagné was hired as a teacher of English and started in September 1954. The school board minutes trace his Inuktitut adventure. In February 1955, "it was reported that arrangements would be made to record on magnetic tape certain lessons in the Eskimo language; these readings would be made by Eskimos in the Sanatorium in some instances and in others it was expected that a person in the employ of the Department in Ottawa would be able to assist us."[165] In addition, the school principal, George Young, was to make a trip to the Charles Camsell to observe teaching methods, if the Indian Health Services paid. Whether he went or not is not indicated elsewhere. *The Camsell Mosaic: The Charles Camsell Hospital, 1945–1985* has a section on the hospital school, but is silent on the question of language.

In April 1956, about twenty months after Gagné appeared on the scene, he was reported giving a luncheon presentation on "a text book he was preparing for use by Eskimos." This was followed by an "informal discussion of the problems attendant upon the presence of so many Eskimos in the institution. R. Gagné and Mr. Young explained that much new ground had to be broken and that all work with Eskimos was of an experimental nature."[166] In June, Gagné had liaised with Northern Affairs and was taking suggestions toward a new draft. He planned also to take a course in linguistics at the Université de Montréal over the summer, with emphasis on Inuktitut.[167] While Gagné was gone, his primer was put into use, for the *Hamilton Spectator* reported in September that "John Dowding, who normally teaches at Robert Land School, spent the past summer with a group of young Eskimos at the Mountain Sanatorium."[168] This information appeared below a photograph of Dowding at the blackboard, with a pupil who was being asked to write, in syllabic script, the Inuktitut translation of "the man has a fish." Below was reproduced a "sample page from Canada's first Eskimo-English primer, *The Life of Makpa*," with text by Gagné, illustrations by Jane Morgan. Phrases were provided in three versions: English, Inuktitut syllabic and Inuktitut in the Roman alphabet. The main purpose, Gagné explained, was to teach English, "but we also want them to be able to read and write their own language. Some of these children come here as mere babies, they have been away from home for several years, and now they must have some means of communicating with their parents. The only way they can do that is by learning the Eskimo syllabics."[169]

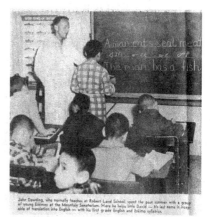

A child at the blackboard in a Mountain Sanatorium schoolroom. © *Hamilton Spectator*, September 12, 1956. Courtesy of the Archives of HHS & FHS, 1980.1.70.21.1.

Supplementing the primer were Inuktitut lessons over the San PA system each morning. A Hamilton branch of Remington Rand produced a syllabics typewriter that was in use at the San. An

163

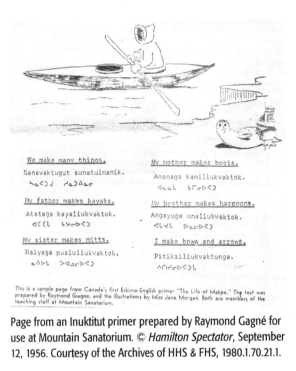

We make many things.
Sanavaktugut sunatuinanik.
ᔃᕐᑦᒍᑦ ᒃᑕᓴᒃᑯ

My father makes kayaks.
Atataga kayaliukvaktok.
ᐊᑕᑕ ᑲᔭᓕᑯ

My sister makes mitts.
Naiyaga pualuliukvaktok.
ᓇᐃᔭ ᑉᕿᑯᕐᑎ

My mother makes boots.
Ananaga kamiliukvaktok.
ᐊᓇᓇ ᑲᒥᓕᑯᕐᑎ

My brother makes harpoons.
Angayuga unaliukvaktok.
ᐊᖓᔪ ᐅᓇᓕᑯᕐᑎ

I make bows and arrows.
Pitiksiliukvaktunga.
ᐱᑎᒃᓯᓕᑯᕐᑐᖓ

This is a sample page from Canada's first Eskimo-English primer "The Life of Makpa." The text was prepared by Raymond Gagne, and the illustrations by Miss Jane Morgan. Both are members of the teaching staff at Mountain Sanatorium.

Page from an Inuktitut primer prepared by Raymond Gagné for use at Mountain Sanatorium. © *Hamilton Spectator*, September 12, 1956. Courtesy of the Archives of HHS & FHS, 1980.1.70.21.1.

Inuktitut essay-writing contest drew two hundred entries. Revisions to the primer were ongoing.[170]

This was an important moment, seeming to signal a turn away from the insistence on total immersion in English and the devaluation and even direct suppression of Aboriginal languages that darkened the days of many residential school-children. But it is not possible to judge how long-lived this particular experiment was, nor how intensive the schooling. After all, language is gestural and contextual, and so best learned in the uses of everyday life, rather than in a primer-and-classroom situation. Also, there were several dialects at the San, since the patients came from all over the Eastern Arctic and Northern Quebec, so the Inuktitut language being taught must have been rudimentary, and perhaps rather arbitrary. Standard written Inuktitut did not yet exist – and indeed Gagné ultimately made it his mission to elaborate a modernized, pan-Arctic tongue for a modernizing people, from which could grow an Inuit literature. Explicit comparison with the linguistic situation of Greenlanders, as well as with that of the French-speaking Québécois, became the bud from which emerged Inuit authority over language use in Nunavut and Nunavik. If language was to be maintained and vocabulary enlarged, then some mechanism for preserving it and arresting language shift, while still facilitating bilingualism, had to be developed, and only an Inuit authority could claim the necessary legitimacy. In fact, as of 2014 this project was still ongoing.

Since the object at the San in 1956 was to improve communications with home, rather than language capacity per se, this effort was probably displaced by tape recording.[171] Eight months later Principal Young reported to the board "on various aspects of the work with Eskimos . . . Provision of teaching material for these people was being slowly developed. It was now being attempted to provide outside reading for the Eskimos in their own language . . . The Principal asked if, in view of the relatively short time in which Eskimos would be at the sanatorium in great numbers, more experimentation was justified."[172] In December 1957 Gagné took a leave of absence and was not expected back until May. Meanwhile the Inuit children were making rapid progress in English, but the board hired Johnny Eksinak as an interpreter on a twelve-month contract to begin in September. He arrived earlier, but left early as well, in March 1958. While in Hamilton he co-edited, with a Joanasie of Cape Dorset[173] (perhaps Salamonie), a magazine in syllabics. Called *Northern Lights and Shadows*, copies of this production were distributed to HBC posts by the *Howe*.

Among the adults at the San a Dick and Jane English reader was in use, as appeared in a photograph of a patient on bedrest studying his copy, but attempts were made to provide Inuktitut and Cree reading material in the patient newsletter. Unfortunately, issues beyond 1955 are not archived. If and when these are found, they will perhaps provide a link to *Northern Lights and Shadows*, and this in turn to *Inuktitut*, which would establish the sanatorium root of secular literature in Inuktitut.

The nurses could escape the uncertainties of the educators and administrators by treating the patients with loving care, especially when the patient was very young. They knew just what to do, and knew it so surely that they might do it even when it was forbidden: a nurse might climb up on the bed to comfort a mournful child for a while, which was definitely not allowed. But tenderness and consistent attention, though essential, are of course insufficient. True compassion wants to be lastingly effective, wants the other to thrive and grow; and effectiveness requires knowledge. If a child has tuberculosis or leukemia, we cannot love the disease away, it must be *reasoned* away – that is, the cause and cure of the disease must be learned. Euro-Canadians had knowledge of tuberculosis – the disease, its agent and its cure – in part. But of Vallee's questions, only one – "What can be done to render the effects of hospitalization less disruptive?" – was answered, and that not until 1957, when a social welfare worker went on the EAP. The principal question – "What can be done to take fullest advantage of the 'captive' situation to engender desireable social and psychological changes?" – was not.[174] Nobody really knew and time ran out; that is, the drugs subdued the microbe and the captivity ended. The problem of converting patronage on both sides to something resembling partnership shifted to the expanding settlements in the Inuit homeland. There, from within a new set of constraints, a new generation began around 1970 to propose their own answers.

5.

The archives of Hamilton Health Sciences hold a great many photographs of unidentified Inuit patients. These are in the form of contact sheets struck from a cache of negatives found in a cabinet in a disused laboratory. Each of the dozens of sheets contains about twenty images, which formed the basis of an oral history project conducted in Pangnirtung, one of many centres where people assembled before going south (Cowall).

Whenever a group of patients was scheduled to return home from the San, photographs of those remaining in care would be taken to send with the returneees to show friends and relatives back home that those still at the San were, if not entirely well, at least properly cared for, and in good cheer. And indeed, many of those photographed are smiling broadly and posing diligently. Some illustrated their well-being by dressing the scene with a carving they had made. One woman held her math notebook. Others were clearly not feeling well at all, whether owing to the disease or to the drugs they were taking, and were simply lying abed, inert and exhausted. Still others were sitting up or even out of bed altogether, but looked quite miserable. The occasion had evidently turned their thoughts toward home, and so saddened them that they were unable to muster the emotional strength to conceal

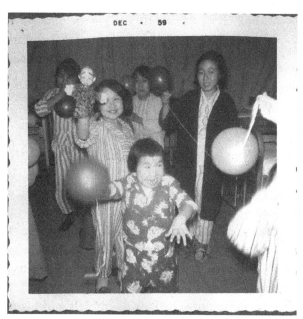

Party at the Holbrook Pavilion, Mountain Sanatorium.
© Eka Berends, private collection.

their misery. Or perhaps they had recently undergone some undignified or distressing procedure that had left them subdued and unhappy. The discomfort and anxiety of the treatments and the various diagnostic procedures found expression in the doggerel verse and comic essays that, interspersed with gossipy banter from the wards, made up the bulk of the patient-produced newsletter that was a therapeutic staple at every large sanatorium.

Mountain Views, the "voice of Santown," was the version circulated at Mountain Sanatorium. It was produced by the radio department, logically enough, as an extension of its educational and entertainment functions. A typical issue contained, along with burlesques and cartoons meant to make light of what was difficult to bear but had nonetheless to be borne, an article of medical popularization by one of the doctors on staff. The Cree and Inuit patients no doubt had much the same response to the drugs and the same experience of x-ray, bronchoscopy and the rest, so the mimeograph literature can be drawn on to describe the kind of thing that had to be endured.

First of all the enforced rest and confinement were hard for some to abide, especially those who resented their position of dependence and subordination. In 1957 Josephine Chaisson, a professor of social work at the University of Toronto, was hired to study *Irregular Discharges from Ontario Sanatoria*. She found that by that date, some patients viewed treatment primarily as chemotherapy, and thought they could just as well take the drugs at home as in a sanatorium. Others rejected bedrest because of the troubling dependency. It relieved patients of responsibility to perform, but not necessarily of worry about those responsibilities. "Feelings of inadequacy, shame and guilt may become so intolerable for these patients that they will be unable to follow treatment to maximum benefit," she wrote (Chaisson, 24). Then there was the fact that "Bed Rest may provide a patient with unwelcome opportunities to look at himself and his past behaviour" (ibid., 24). Some didn't like the noise on the wards, or the continual gossip; others chafed under childish rules enforced by nurses perceived as patronizing martinets. Among the four hundred in the "study universe," some also complained about the forced cohabitation with "New Canadians, Eskimos, Indians" (ibid., 18).

Going AWOL was not much of a possibility for unilingual Inuit thousands of kilometres from familiar ground, but one did choose it. In 1951 David Mikeyook walked out of Mountain Sanatorium and vanished for seven weeks. The limestone face of the Niagara Escarpment to which the San grounds extended was, and still is, a jumble of steep drops and wooded slopes, broken by several waterfalls. Mikeyook's corpse was found on the bank of a stream by kids out for a hike. The verdict of the eventual coroner's inquest was that the death was the result of an "unlawful escape"; actually, as the editors of the *Globe and Mail* reminded their readers, the man had starved to death. The notion that someone brought south to be helped had then died of apparent neglect was infuriating to some. Accusations of hypocrisy and racism flew thick and fast. How could someone go missing in an urban area for seven weeks and not be found? Had anyone been looking? J. David Ford of Port Hope wrote to say that "many inquiries were made about David Mikeyook on my last trip to the Arctic . . . As is my custom I explained in detail that he was being looked after with the greatest care . . . I have seen many a white man hopelessly lost. I have also seen the feverish and hasty search parties organized in a few minutes by the Eskimos to save a life at great peril to their own, for is he not a stranger?"[175] A nurse with some Arctic time on her CV observed that

> the authorities will say that the poor man was infectious and therefore he could not go back [north]. Why couldn't he? Why else was that $4 million hospital built up on James Bay? . . . It is a handsome hospital even though it does seem to come closer to being a magnificent sepulchre where we could at last lay to rest our national conscience which had become a bit smelly with the neglect to these races for a few hundred years . . . Doctors, we nurses, and the clergy still like to be told that we do 'noble' work. And the whole lot of us – and all the rest of the public – let a sick and lonely man crawl away and die. A Merry Christmas to all of us.[176]

During the initial weeks or months of rest, the patient was served up the inevitable strep course. Not every nurse was equally skilled in giving the injections, which were vaguely humiliating, and there were odd side effects, described as follows by one bemused patient in a 1949 issue of the newsletter of Saskatchewan's Fort Qu'Appelle Sanatorium:

> The reactions to strep in the first week
> Have a taste rather bitter-sweet;
> Since there's a little gall in every cup
> We drink it in to "Bottoms Up!"
>
> It affects people in different ways
> As for myself, I was in a daze
> But some go crazy, others just eat
> Others don't do anything but sleep.[177]

The para-aminosalicylic that came with the strep was no treat either:

I tossed around and restlessly I gazed up at the moon,
I swear I heard the devil say, "Cheer up, I'll see you soon."
My stomach felt on fire, it was a burning mess,
I called the nurse, she said to me, "It's just the P.A.S."[178]

Sainty Morris, in his youth a TB patient at Nanaimo Indian Hospital, told the story of his experience there to Professor Laurie Drees:

Being in the hospital was something I was not used to. Right away they started me on needles, and every morning I got a needle in my hip. I was so pockmarked from the needles that they would switch to my other hip and switch back. They had a medication which they called PAS. It was a yellow liquid, bitter tasting, but I got used to it. Then they changed it to another form of PAS in the colour of vanilla. When I think about it now, it makes me wonder. When they put me on the first drug it was as if they were "trying out" things on me, like they were experimenting. (quoted in Drees, xxvii)

Strep could not be avoided, but some of the pills could be dodged. Hence the need for a little no-nonsense talk from time to time.

How many times have you or your fellow patients on the ward beefed about those P.A.S. pills? How many times have you consigned them to the water closet and not your stomach? Just a few occasions huh? Well let me tell you, Friend, those P.A.S. pills are not handed out to you to play "Let's hit the squirrel," but for a definite purpose . . . Where streptomycin has been given alone, it was found 80 to 90 percent of cases became resistant to the drug by the end of three months . . . However P.A.S. . . . caused the resistance rate to drop to 15 percent or even as low as 5 percent in some cases. And this state of affairs could be carried out for 12 or 18 months without resistance developing . . . Hundreds of tuberculous patients who would be unable to benefit from streptomycin alone, have been able to take it for long periods and that in fact alone, probably meant that their lives were saved. If you fall in that category, I think you'll agree a little indigestion and occasional nausea is worth having.[179]

Once a patient had been taken under care, the lab undertook to answer questions that would guide treatment. Was the individual's disease in fact tuberculosis? Or was something else going on? If the TB bacillus was present, was it the human variety (as distinct from the bovine or avian)? Was there any other micro-organism involved? If TB was not the pathogen, then what was? If TB was the principal agent of the patient's illness, then was the strain resistant to any of the drugs in use? To gauge this last the bug was cultured, then the crop exposed to the drugs. Around 1952 seven thousand cultures a year were set at Mountain San, which implies that the seven hundred fifty patients were being checked on average every six weeks or so. A culture had to be barren for eight weeks before it was deemed negative. X-ray films sufficed to show that the disease was not progressing, but could not detect small bacteria-sheltering foci that could recolonize the patient, so several cultures were checked before the apparently cured were released. In pulmonary disease these questions were answered by testing the bronchial secretions and, less frequently, the pleural/chest fluid. The method by which the necessary sample was collected could be quite uncomfortable.

In health, the mucosa of the lung continually produce a slightly viscous fluid that is moved upward by ciliated cells to the larynx, where it is unconsciously swallowed. Irritated mucosa increase their output, and this increase may be swallowed or expectorated. The expectorate can be revealing, but is more often simply confusing, since it may contain sloughed skin cells, a variety of bacteria and bits of material that have accumulated in the nose, mouth and throat. A better specimen can be had by swabbing the throat, provoking a spasmodic cough and catching the product of the cough on the swab. Even better is a sample obtained by gastric lavage, that is, from the stomach. This was the preferred means with children, who tended to swallow rather than spit. The procedure however was not fun. The patient had to fast, and then put up with the insertion of a hose down the throat to tap the stomach contents. Harry Rubin described the experience for the *L.A. Sanscript*, and it was reprinted in *Mountain Views* sometime in 1950.

> I'm sick to my stomick clear down to my toes
> From trying to swallow that little red hose.
> It's the gol durndest feelin'; I choked and I gagged
> While those durn little bugs refused to be snagged.
> "Now just take it easy," said nurse, "and don't squirm."
> Did she ever swallow a seven foot worm?
> So back down my throat she would run that old hose,
> And just where it stopped the Lord only knows.[180]

Nasty as it was, at least one was awake and aware for the gastric lavage. Bronchoscopy however was conducted with the subject in a twilight state and unfolded like a bad dream. A sequence of photographs taken at the Mountain San begins in mid-story, with the patient, a grown man and not small, hanging three-quarters off the gurney in the arms of staff. Involved were Ellen Ewart, someone who may have been Dr. Yang and a third handler. They were catching the patient as Dr. Rabinowitz bent and turned to follow along with the already inserted instrument as the patient flung himself around. After a few more wild contortions, the poor scopee finally succumbed to the anaesthetic, and came to rest in a workable posture. It is not possible to tell if the instrument in use was a bronchoscope proper or a laryngoscope, but it was probably the former. The bronchoscope at that date was quite rigid. The doctor had to negotiate the larynx, then advance and withdraw the scope in order to examine each airway. This uncomfortable process was difficult for the gagging patient to tolerate, so they were first sedated and then the larynx itself numbed. The technique allowed very precise localization and sampling of diseased tissue.

In addition to this sort of episode, the chafing constraint and ennui of bedrest, and the blurring side effects of the drugs, there was the odd moment of high emotion when a taped message recorded by parents or siblings back home would be played.[181]

Hello my son, I do love you, we are listening to your message on the record. I want you to listen and do as you're told to do by the nurses and doctors. Your brother and your Mom, we are very happy to hear your voice . . . Your mom came home from the South not long ago, she was quite sick for a while but she's home and well again . . . I'm not quite sure of what to say for now so I'll say bye for now. (Tester, McNicoll and Irniq, 135)

6.

The fullest personal account of the experience of an Inuk at Mountain Sanatorium is a scant six or seven pages. It is that of Minnie Aodla Freeman and appears in her memoir of growing up motherless in the James Bay region in the mid-twentieth century. Supplementing these few pages are recollections provided orally to Alexandra Grygier in 1988, and relayed in *A Long Way from Home*.

Approached from the Euro-Canadian side, Aodla Freeman's is a coming-of-age story within which can be recognized another familiar genre, the captivity narrative – but with a twist. This form, as Linda Colley explains in her broad survey, *Captives: Britain, Empire and the World*, arose in English literature as a consequence of the audacity of underequipped British marauders who ventured into others people's lands, and mainly recounts the experience of Europeans in the hands of captors in Africa, America, Afghanistan, et cetera. The reverse also occurred, leaving far fewer records. Colley identifies the form as the germ of *Robinson Crusoe* and *Gulliver's Travels*. As to Aodla Freeman's models, one would have to inquire of the author herself; however the experience of captivity is certainly what she describes. She speaks of being "kidnapped" to school, and visited there by her father and grandfather, but not redeemed. "I am sure they had come to take me home, but I guess they had no ransom" (Aodla Freeman, 107).

Born in 1937 to seventeen-year-old parents, Aodla Freeman lost her mother at the age of four and was raised by her paternal grandparents in the absence of her father, who was often away working. Against the objections of her grandmother, Aodla Freeman was placed in residence at St. Thomas Anglican School in Moose Factory, where she passed two years as the lone Inuk among two hundred girls, mostly Cree speakers. The third year she spent on the land with her father and grandparents, before returning, again over the protests of her grandmother, to school, this time to the Catholic establishment at Fort George, along with a number of her cousins. (She was strictly forbidden by her Anglican family to convert to Catholicism.) This pattern continued with a year at school and a year in the country. During her next stint away, she was set to work, for five dollars a month, at the hospital, and encouraged to become a nurse. Her tasks were demanding. During the late winter of 1952 she became fatigued. A chest x-ray turned up a spot on one lung, and she was taken to the convent hospital at Moosonee, with its train connection to southern Canada, and then transferred to the better-equipped Moose Factory hospital nearby. From there she went on to Hamilton with seven others, all of whom received a speedy diagnosis while she continued to wait for the doctors to pronounce. Meanwhile she kept busy by translating for the medical staff as they communicated with the Inuit and Cree who had come south with her.

> My *qallunaat* roommates began to urge me to ask when I would get needles like everybody else, to find out what was wrong with me. It is your body, they would say, and you have a right to know. The cultural beliefs that I was raised with and their urgings began to get mixed in my mind. My culture told me not to ask, that in this situation I might cause the people who were taking care of me to alter their behaviour completely, that I should accept what was happening and not force the hands that held my destiny. I figured that they would tell me when they were ready. I was X-rayed again, blood samples were taken, and the questions asked once more. Did I have such a complicated sickness that they did not know what to do with me? Finally, I was told that I had a spot on my left lung. I had known that at Fort George. It was not serious, but it was

enough to put me to bed. I began to get needles. I dreaded
them. Some nurses did not hurt, but others gave needles that
sent pain all the way down my leg. (Aodla Freeman, 175)

The brevity of this account both requires and sharply limits
interpretation. Judging from the rest of her book, it is unlikely that
Aodla Freeman has omitted anything out of delicacy. Elsewhere she
is quite candid about personal matters, physical and emotional. The
length of the delay in commencing treatment is not specified, so
the reader is left to guess at the reasons. The doctors may have been
attempting to confirm a diagnosis of TB by cultivating the organism
from sputum or some other materials. (X-ray alone was not always
conclusive. An exchange of letters kept on file at Weston compares
the accuracy of diagnoses made by two physicians on the 1962 EAP.
In tagging active tuberculosis, they were both right about half the
time. Inactive TB or some other disease accounted for the rest.) They
may also have been puzzling over a couple of other items in her file: a
mysterious seizure – mysterious to white doctors, but known to Inuit
and Cree, who called it *ocheepitoko*, the pulling sensation, in which
tingling and weakness may be followed by the painless contraction of
the muscles of a foot. This seizure, and a long hiatus following first
menses, which caused the good sisters at Fort George considerable
alarm when fourteen-year-old Minnie mentioned it to them, may
have caused the doctors to hesitate. As it was still early days in the
San's transactions with Inuit and other First Nations patients, the
clinicians may also have been waiting to see the response of her aunts
to streptomycin, since, if the single lung spot was the whole of her
pathology, Aodla Freeman had only a mild case.

What did not occur, however, was any meaningful conversation
between the patient – who had already acquired some nursing
experience herself, including textbook instruction in anatomy – and
the San staff. This state of affairs persisted for some time. According
to Aodla Freeman, "I asked one day if I could be up and around more,
since I had to be up all the time to translate in the different rooms. The
answer was no, I could not, as I might cause my lung to worsen. I could
not understand that, why I would get worse if I walked a little more

and strained my brain a little more when I translated. Yes, we were shipped like cargo and meant to behave like cargo" (Aodla Freeman, 176).

Strep was evidently given on alternate days, or perhaps every third day, and unaccompanied. As PAS was in use, but was generally offered as a licorice- or wintergreen-flavoured drink and taken at least once daily, Aodla Freeman would have remembered had she received it. The combination of PAS and streptomycin was under study from 1948 at Weston, and the results were published in 1950: the pairing did not clear the microbe any more effectively than did strep alone; but it did greatly reduce the production of strep-resistant bacilli. This is a strong recommendation, so its absence from Aodla Freeman's treatment plan is puzzling. Isoniazid was still in the wings – Aodla Freeman had been slightly too early for it. In the late spring or summer of 1952, her shots were stopped, and she and her two aunts were permitted outdoor exercise.

> A couple of months after our arrival, we were all moved to another building. We were put in one big room. There were eight of us, my two aunts, five *qallunaat* women, and myself. We all got to know each other. The *qallunaat* women were always visited by their relatives, and these too we got to know . . .
>
> Christmas came and went. I was knitting a lot, while my aunts were kept busy making Inuit dolls and parkas. Sometimes I stuffed the dolls for one of my aunts. Most of the time I was bored, and wondered what I could really do. Teachers came around . . . but permission had to be granted by the doctors if a patient wanted to take on an extra project. I got my permission, and took grade nine and ten in math, spelling and history. Now I was busy, ready to please my teacher who came around every week to see my work. All of us were doing something, one was taking art lessons, one was knitting, one who was from Yugoslavia took English. (Aodla Freeman, 177)

When her aunts went home, Aodla Freeman was prevailed upon to remain as a translator, and went to live in the nurses' residence. She was assigned to the children's ward – this would have been the Holbrook Pavilion, which opened in December 1951 – and began again to train as a nurse. She struggled with this choice, but stayed in southern Canada out of compassion for those who were entering this unfamiliar and disconcerting situation. She was certainly needed. In the summer of 1953 she went to Mount Hope Airport (now John C. Munro Hamilton International Airport) to translate for a group of Inuit arrivals. The plane smelled strongly of uncured sealskin and full diapers, and everyone was apprehensive and disoriented. Registration was long, and the partitioning of patients by age and gender was upsetting, especially for women who were separated from infants or young children.[182]

Though frequently called upon for her skills, Aodla Freeman continued to be estranged from her putative colleagues. She made no close friend, nor, she says, did she try, as she regarded her situation as temporary. Consequently when her father sent word that he wished her to return home immediately, she was unable to confide the real reason to her disappointed superior: that she had been betrothed since infancy, and that her prospective husband's mother felt it was high time for the marriage to begin (Aodla Freeman, 180). Aodla Freeman's place as translator seems to have been taken by Aniapik Witaltuk, who came from Moosonee in October 1954, and perhaps Mary Panigusiq, who was there by August 1955 when her name appears in the patient newsletter. Also there around this time was Ann Koolatalik (later Padlo). From 1952 on there were always one or more Inuktitut speakers, either translators or health care trainees, among the staff.

Aodla Freeman passed through the San at the beginning of the chemo era, responded well to the standard treatment of sanatorium routine plus streptomycin, got better and does not mention any relapses in her memoir. Although she was often unhappy, disliked confinement and was socially isolated, she bore up and did her duty as she had been raised to do on the land.

Less fortunate was Maggie Hatuk, an aide with the medical team during the *Howe*'s 1958 tour. Hatuk, a native of Kangirsuk in Nunavik, was among the first Inuit to be sent south, arriving at Weston in 1945 at the age of eight for treatment that went on for two years. There she underwent surgery with spinal fusion. In 1947 she was the cover girl (lace on her collar and bows in hair) for the fiftieth yearbook of the National Sanatorium Association. The accompanying copy, evidently addressed to any children made curious by the cover, was the epitome of a captivity narrative.

> Maggie is a little Eskimo girl from Baffin Land. Many wonderful things have happened to her. She had a ride in an aeroplane. She was placed in a soft bed so different from her rug. There were mostly little white boys and girls in the big place to which she was taken. Many of them could not walk and run either. They smiled and talked to her, but she could only understand the smiles until she later learned the strange language of the white man . . .
>
> Then one day the men and women in white paid extra attention to her. They told her she was to have a long sleep and while she was asleep they would do something for her back which, after a little while, would make her strong and straight . . .
>
> When she woke up she was sick and filled with pain. She could not move because she had a stone dress on . . . How happy she was when they took the stone dress off . . . Then one day, the most wonderful thing happened to Maggie. The nurses brought her the prettiest dress in all the world. It had blue, and red and pink strings worked in a pattern that even Maggie's mother, who was the best sewer on the tribe, could not have done. She was so happy, she nearly cried, and when they gave her shiny, black slippers, she did cry.[183]

Hatuk had TB of the spine and evidently there was damage to vertebrae or to one or more of the spinal disks, which could lead to spinal deformity or pain during motion. In such a case it was helpful to remove moribund tissue and fuse adjacent vertebrae by placing many bits of bone graft between them. The bone was usually taken from the patient's own pelvis, and provided scaffolding for further bone to grow upon, as well as osteoblasts (bone-growing cells) and ready-to-use proteins. Such surgery might also involve the implantation of steel pins, rods and screws, audacities pioneered by Fritz Lange shortly after 1900 for treatment of spinal deformities in tuberculosis, and revived in the forties to deal with conditions resulting from polio. Post-operatively the patient was placed in a cast to reduce the demands on the affected parts, and presumably given a course of antibiotics to kill the bacillus. However, immobilization following surgery imposed its own costs: loss of strength and connective tissue mass, and a consequent reduction of the range of motion. Loss of ankle strength, for example, led to foot drop, a disorder of the gait in which the toes cannot be lifted to initiate a step. This could be averted in someone who was lying on their back by placing sandbags at their soles, to prevent the muscles from losing their normal lengths. When the patient resumed walking, braces were used to supplement the connective tissues in maintaining correct alignments.

By 1958, when she would have been twenty, Hatuk was recruited to the *Howe*, but had still not recovered much of her native tongue; nor was she ever fully cured. In May 1963 she was admitted to Weston with a diagnosis of miliary tuberculosis, and stayed until December.[184] According to a cousin Imaapik (also known as Jacob Partridge), in the mid-sixties Hatuk was living at Iqaluit, as she had to be near a "comprehensive medical facility for what she ended up with after her hospitalization in Toronto," and here she died "due to medication she became allergic to."[185]

The record of a Cree woman from James Bay who was treated to the entire repertoire of available techniques – sanatorium routine, triple drug chemo and restorative surgery – has been preserved at Weston as a sample for the benefit of eventual students. The folder of charts and reports provides details of close combat with the disease and of what was going on inside these widely spaced buildings with the broad lawns and the well-tended flower beds.

X, let's call her, is identified as a housewife who entered the Moose Factory hospital in June 1953, age twenty-nine. She was there for a year before being sent on to Muskoka, and thence transferred to Weston in August 1954. This woman had mild pulmonary TB and a serious infection in one hip, which had brought her into the hospital. The end of the femur, normally held into the acetabulum (the socket of the hip bone), had been structurally altered and no longer had the rigidity of bone. This had caused deformation owing to the loss of proper anchorage for muscles. By the time she got to Weston, the lung disease had been knocked down by chemotherapy, and the deformity corrected by immobilization and traction. However, the disintegrating, or punky, end of the femur was riding directly on the ilium, reducing the apparent length of her leg by about seven centimetres, even though the actual loss of bone was only about three centimetres.

The surgeons at Weston proposed to partially reconstruct this hip joint by pulling the bone down and away from the pelvis, and filling the gap with a bone graft. On August 20, X was fitted with a Steinmann pin, a length of steel that was inserted at a nick in the skin just above the knee, and turned through the end of the femur by means of a hand drill, then on through and out the other side of the limb. Pulleys were mounted to each end of the pin, in preparation to receive a stirrup. Cable linked the stirrup over pulleys to weights that, over the course of weeks, drew the bone away from the pelvis. Next, on October 21, the doctors operated to clean up the infected bone end and socket. After the musculature was laid aside, the hip joint capsule was partly exposed, at which point "some white curdy material" appeared. This was removed, the joint capsule opened and cleared of more of the same, and then punky tissue removed from the end of the femur and the inside of the hip socket. Consequently, when the head of the femur was realigned with the socket, there was a gap. This was plugged with bone taken from X's pelvis.[186]

At this juncture it was sometimes the practice to cut clean through the femur, at a point high up near the head, in order to eliminate the leverage of the long bone during the time it took the hip to set. By the time the severed ends of the femur grew back together, the hip too would be fused and strong enough to withstand the restored leverage (Frederick R. Thompson).

After everything was put back together and the wounds closed up and dressed, the patient's leg and body were encased in a plaster cast. By then she had been anaesthetized for more than two and half hours, and was on her fourth flask of blood.

The end result of this procedure would be to fuse the remnant head of the femur and the hip bone, so as to keep the femur from drifting around. However, the missing bone would cause that leg to shorten, so a second operation was undertaken on May 6, about seven months after the first. This time the upper end of the bone was sliced obliquely but not parted, so as to make a hinge. The bone was then moved on the hinge to a better angle with respect to the hip, and the resulting gap at the hinge filled with a wedge of bone again taken from the pelvis. Again a cast was put on to hold everything in place while the tissues knit. By November, X was up and moving around with the support of a walker. In January she went home, with the left leg only slightly shorter than the other, but with restricted motion of the left knee. (This was the Catch-22 of these operations – the cast immobilized the knee to protect the work on the hip, but immobilizing the knee caused loss of function.) By then she had been at Weston for five hundred twenty-three days

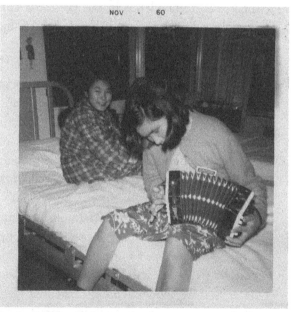

Passing the time at Mountain Sanatorium.
© Eka Berends, private collection.

– about a year and a half, on top of the time already spent at Moose Factory and Muskoka.

The era of long stays was drawing to an end for all but surgical cases like these.[187] Already in 1954 Weston was treating some of the locals on an outpatient basis. The domiciliary approach was slower in coming for the Inuit however, for reasons that have not been spelled out. The rapid decline in resident numbers at the end of the 1950s seems to indicate that recalcitrant pulmonary, renal or bone cases were scarce. The patient load was strongly shifted away from Hamilton in 1961, with the transfer of fifty-eight to Clearwater. Le Pas was a long way to go for treatment that might as well be given at Hamilton, or at Weston in Toronto, but it may have been a stage on the way home rather than a long-term change of hospital. Weston, as the new centre for Ontario, welcomed thirteen patients evacuated by the EAP from Arctic Bay and other Baffin communities in September 1962.[188] The tone of correspondence in the Weston archives gives the impression that the administration responded dutifully rather than happily to their new assignment.

By the end of 1963 there were about one hundred Inuit (and seven hundred others) at the hospital, and a number of Inuit out of proportion to their representation in the patient population were flouting the rules – so persistently that C. A. Wicks, the superintendent, drafted a letter of complaint to Moore. Wicks reminded Moore of all the hospital had done to encourage compliance, making craft work possible at almost any hour on the ward or in the workshop; enlisting the help of Bishop Marsh, as well as of Betty Marwood and her interpreter, to make everything clear in Inuktitut; and circulating photos and taped messages, including those provided by the Inuit service of the CBC. Nonetheless, adult patients persisted in leaving the grounds to visit shops and restaurants in the neighbourhood. Wicks therefore reiterated his understanding that the department would remove promptly anyone whom the super requested to be removed. However, the heart of the problem, Wicks repeated, was that the department had yet to arrange, as he had urged a year before, for non-infectious patients to leave the hospital and continue on chemo in some other situation at some other place.[189]

By February of 1965 the numbers at Weston were down to forty, and Moore advised the hospital that for the foreseeable future, accommodation for about thirty a year would meet the department's needs. Meanwhile Northern Affairs initiated the McGill-Baffin program to link the new general hospital at Iqaluit with the McGill University hospitals. Air travel to Baffin was by way of Dorval. The next year, the Montreal Children's Hospital began sending a resident to the Iqaluit hospital each month. This reduced evacuations and provided follow-up for returnees. The new sedentary life was hard on children, who suffered from increased occurrence of impetigo, myopia, dental cavities and frequent long-lasting ear infections (Baxter, 91–95). TB cases resident in southern Canada kept shrinking in numbers, but even in 1970 there were patients at Weston. One of these, Peter Ittinuar (later the first Inuit member of Parliament), along with Joanne Mucktar, made the syllabic translation of the outpatient instructions to the homeward bound.[190]

> The most important thing about treatment is to start if away from home in a hospital, and after you come home, to take the medicine (pills) <u>every day</u> for <u>two years</u> . . . It is because the T.B. germs are very tough, it takes long time to kill them . . . members of the family or friends should remind you to take the pills . . . You do not forget your hunting equipment when you go hunting, so do not forget your ammunition (the T.B. pills) when your body is still busy killing the T.B. germs inside your body.

FIVE: SEQUELAE

1.

In 1949 a local woman named Gladys McAndrew was asked to visit one Inuit and three Cree women who had recently arrived in Hamilton. She did so, and continued to go by the wards twice a week for the next twelve years. She also saw returning patients off at the train station or the airport. Childless, McAndrew had two Inuit girls as her house guests while they were in school. (She had herself been a teacher, and her husband was head of modern languages at Westdale Secondary School.) McAndrew's involvement at the San was a development of her work with the supply department of Anglican missionary services. The Dorcas Society, of which she was diocesan secretary treasurer from 1935 on, and later national secretary for a term, organized Anglican women in support of the missions. The Dorcas sisters arranged the purchase or collection of clothing for residential schools and mission stations, sometimes finding it cheaper to sew the garments themselves. McAndrew was in effect a volunteer medical welfare worker, and even accompanied patients back to James Bay and escorted others south.[191]

Commenting for Sivertz on a report about the situation on the Belcher Islands in 1953, Graham Rowley noted that visits from prospectors were increasing and that some of these white men left "a good deal to be desired." As there were no RCMP officers or missionaries there, and the HBC post manager was Inuit, Rowley believed "the Belchers would be an ideal place to station a white man for an extended period to help and guide the natives in adapting themselves to conditions which change there very rapidly. It should preferably be a young man who intends to devote his life to Eskimo administration."[192] In other words, a sort of lay missionary employed by the Canadian state rather than a church. As a self-recruited helper McAndrew anticipated, as did several others, the emerging role of northern service officer, not officially established until 1956.

Just as McAndrew issued from the Anglican Church, Alex Spalding came out of the Hudson's Bay Company and Terry Ryan from the weather service. Even the RCMP produced one of these enthusiasts, in the person of Constable Van Norman, stationed at Iqaluit, who put up a thousand dollars of his own money to expedite the construction of a workshop and display area for carvers in the spring of 1953. This was in anticipation of an organizational visit from artist James Houston, which may or may not have occurred. In reporting Van Norman's zeal to his superior for relay to the deputy minister, Superintendent Larsen mentioned that the constable was himself "something of an artist in painting and photography, and has the ability to make a success of a project of this nature."[193] Sabean, eventually the doctor at Pangnirtung, started at a radio station. Farley Mowat was at first a biologist in the Keewatin region of what is now Nunavut. R. G. Williamson, who was in Pangnirtung around the time that Van Norman was active in Iqaluit, was an amateur collector of folklore before studying to become an anthropologist and then hiring on with Northern Affairs as an officer in the Whale Cove and Keewatin regions.

Something similar occurred among the Inuit at this time, facilitated or accelerated by the evacuations. But whereas some of the experienced white enthusiasts were recruited to Robertson's new cadre system, Inuit who had acquired familiarity with Euro-Canadian forms were not, with the possible exception of Abraham Okpik. These persons were employed differently and dubbed, by Frank Vallee, "articulate Eskimos."

Vallee's proposal to document the effects of hospitalization on evacuees had been unsuccessful, but within a few years he was working in the North. At the end of the decade he published some reflections on the determinants of social class at Baker Lake, a community that, like many other Arctic settlements of the day, was newly enlarged by the presence of whites in large numbers, and therefore offered the social scientist "new problems in the social arrangements which one can study as though in a large small-group laboratory" (Vallee, 112). As Vallee saw it, "With the establishment of trading posts, police stations and missions during the early part of this century, a number of new roles were assumed by small numbers of Eskimos; namely the trader's helper, the catechist and the special constable. These people did not realize it, but they were the forerunners of new kinds of groupings for Eskimo society" (ibid., 110). The unfolded result was the division of Inuit society into, roughly, Nunamiut, traditionalists who prefer to live on the land rather than in a settlement, and Kabloonamiut, who prefer the settled life. The members of these groups show mutual respect, but while "successful land people may be admired . . . they are finding it increasingly difficult to find spouses for their sons, there being a tendency for girls on the land to seek a settlement living, and a definite tendency for girls in the settlement to refuse to marry young men on the land, no matter how admired are the families of the young men" (ibid., 121).

There were two other forms of differentiation: by religious denomination and, of a more recent appearance, by age set. Finally, these forms were becoming pan-Arctic, and giving rise to a new consciousness that one could call nationalism, though Vallee, writing in 1962, did not: "Articulate Eskimos are already claiming to speak for all Eskimos *vis à vis* all Kabloona. These articulate Eskimos are Kabloonamiut by our definition and the products of either settlement living or lengthy stays in Kabloona institutions such as hospitals and residential schools. In cultural terms, they are much closer to the Kabloona than they are to the traditional Eskimos. However, for many of them, their identification with the Eskimo reference group is growing increasingly intense. Parallels from the literature on Indians are relevant here" (126).

Who were these "articulate Eskimos" and how much did the sanatoria have to do with their formation? Mountain Sanatorium had been overwhelmed by the sudden loading in of large numbers of students, many of whom had no Euro-Canadian foundation at all – country people suddenly set down in a southern metropolis. However, for a few, who had had some previous schooling, the San seems to have served as an advanced course in Euro-Canadian forms, and these individuals functioned as mediators in parallel with the political cadre fielded by Northern Affairs until both were not so much superseded as simply overtaken and assimilated in the late sixties by a more assertive and activist organizational culture.[194]

When Aodla Freeman was called home by her father after her stay at the San, she realized that she would be unable to please both her father and her nursing supervisor, and chose to satisfy the first – only to find, once home, that her severe and tradition-bound grandmother would not sacrifice her granddaughter's happiness to tradition after all. "In the evening, while brother was out checking our nets, grandmother spoke nervously. 'Minnie, you will never survive with that man. He is too lazy, he will bring nothing from his hunting trips. I have taught you well, not for a lazy man. You will go away and go back to school when the ship arrives'" (Aodla Freeman, 185). Thus Aodla Freeman's elder, whose word commanded her respect, officially designated the white world an acceptable alternative. Aodla Freeman worked for a time as a housekeeper in Moose Factory, then a laundry matron and eventually supervisor of intermediate girls. In 1957 she joined the Department of National Health and Welfare and visited Inuit in hospital. (Probably with Betty Marwood, though Aodla Freeman does not name her colleague.) In 1978 her memoir was published, and in 1981 she became the first director of the Inuit Broadcasting Corporation – meant to offer northern television viewers a choice of Inuit and southern content, because an exclusive diet of the second was thought to be dangerous to the *isuma* of the young.

In Aodla Freeman's recombination of the *Bildungsroman* and the captivity narrative, maturation occurs when, after repeated cycles of captivity and deliverance, two cultures have become mingled in her – or perhaps braided, on the analogy of Michif, with its French noun forms and its Cree verbs. At this point, in a final twist, Aodla Freeman's book becomes a memoir of immigration, which is where she actually begins the telling of it — with her arrival in Ottawa in 1957, aged twenty-one, to take up a position as translator with Northern Affairs. But *immigration* is not quite correct either, though it corresponds to an attitude still espoused by, for instance, Bent Sivertz, and apparently approved by the editor of *North/Nord* as late as 1962. In a mock interview Sivertz, who was of Icelandic origins, declined to write an article on himself as an Icelandic-Canadian, because "the fact of being a Canadian seems to outweigh and render irrelevant all other racial and national connections." To which the editor responded, "Would that apply to Eskimos as well?" Affirmative, said Sivertz.

> On more than one occasion I have suggested to my Eskimo friends that this is the kind of view I hold concerning their status as Eskimos and as Canadians. Their Eskimo ancestry is something I hope they are pleased with and even proud of . . . but it is surprising how rapidly this alters when they start to move freely in this nation. With the passage of even a dozen years the Eskimos I know begin . . . to think along the lines that are the general theme of this conversation. I rather favour this theme, because it seems to me it deals in realities rather than abstractions. It follows a well-known precept . . . "Live in the present." (Sivertz)

Needless to say, this naturalization process has only ever been agreeable to a small minority of Aboriginal persons. Aodla Freeman, although she eventually married on the *qallunaat* side and spent much time in southern Canada, is quite equivocal and insisted on affirming her Aboriginal origins. She wrote, "I have been born twice, once to grow and learn my own culture, and again to learn *qallunaat* culture. Once I was asked which way of life I preferred. I said that I did not really know, and that it would take years to explain my choices and preferences. But it is nice to remember my own ways" (71).

Mary Panigusiq's father, Lazaroosie Kyak, like Aodla Freeman's father, placed great importance on Euro-Canadian schooling for his daughter. As an RCMP special constable at Pond Inlet and Craig Harbour, Kyak arranged with his division commander, Henry Larsen, for Mary to go to school in Hamilton. According to Kenn Harper, an Iqaluit linguist and historian who has been on the scene for thirty years, this was because Kyak hoped that the many Inuit at the San would enable her to keep her language. However, there were rather few Inuit in Hamilton when Mary arrived in 1953, aged fifteen, for a five-year stay. Perhaps it was rather the presence of Ann Koolatalik (later Padlo), the daughter of his brother Panipakoocho hospitalized in 1952, which influenced Kyak's decision. Mary did grades five through eight in Hamilton ("Eskimo in Print").[195] She put her education to use early, acting as an editor and translator for the Inuktitut section of the patient newsletter. In 1956 cousin Ann served as an interpreter on the *Howe*, and by 1958 Mary had become the registrar of the shipborne EAP. Harper says that she took this position during her second tour on the *Howe*, and that she did five in total, although in what capacity he does not specify ("Mary Cousins"). In 1959 however she moved to Ottawa where she worked on *Inuktitut* magazine before being sent to Ghana as a goodwill ambassador in 1963. The next year she married Roger Cousins, a schoolteacher. They went to Grise Fiord where they taught, then in 1967 to Iqaluit and then in 1972 to northern Manitoba. Eventually she took a bachelor of education degree from McGill and finished her working life as a primary school teacher.

Ann meanwhile completed training as a nurse's aide – presumably in 1955 – and then spent a year at St. Luke's in Pangnirtung, before moving on to the Ottawa Civic Hospital, where she became an instructor. Back in the North in 1958 she ran a store in Iqaluit and then signed on with Nordair as a stewardess for a brief stint before being recruited in 1960 to the CBC Northern Service to produce and present *Uqausi*, an Inuktitut language program.[196] By this point she was so familiar with Canadian ways as to have become satirical. Writing to *North/Nord* in 1959 she generously offered guidance for "the Government":

> Please do what I tell you. I know the few things the white people are not supposed to do. Be sure you get up early in the morning. And when you leave to work, watch the traffic, and watch the traffic lights, do not pass the red light. If you finish

work do not go to a party or drink; stay home, be smart, if you get drunk you know you don't know what you're doing. It is no good for your body. Do you understand that? Don't use any more tobacco because this way we often lose a great deal of money. There is another thing, make sure you wash your hands after each meal. Stay home and do nothing else. Please try to be patient, you will be alright. (Padlo)

A similar trajectory was followed by Joanasie Salamonie, who was cured of his TB at Mountain (where his father however died), then returned to continue his schooling before going on to work as a journalist, producer and actor based in Cape Dorset.

Ann Witaltuk, nurse's aide and sometime *Star Weekly* cover girl, also served on the EAP (bringing with her a cousin, Sarah Ekoomiak) before going to work as a stewardess.[197] In 1961 she began dating an Australian-born electrician named Terry Whitfield who was on a job in Great Whale River. This relationship did not last long, but raised a controversy that went all the way to the Supreme Court of Canada. Whitfield's contract contained a no fraternization clause, apparently inserted at the request of Northern Affairs – although when he went to Ottawa to ask the director of Northern Administration about this, he was told that the legality of the proscription was not very sure. (In fact, the clause was an RCAF standing order. Although a civilian, the electrician was working at a military installation, and so his contract indicated that he was subject to the same discipline.)

In any case Whitfield was fired, and he sued. In making his case to the public, via the pages of *North/Nord*, Whitfield offered a new remedy for the presumed danger to naive northern girls posed by the presence of wolves like him. His proposed Act for the Protection of Less Sophisticated Persons was meant to resolve the contradiction between the prohibition of association with Indigenous peoples and the Canadian Bill of Rights. The text of his act, intended as an amendment to the Criminal Code of Canada, created the offence of attempting to "take unfair advantage of any man, woman or child in matters concerning morals, by virtue of one's more sophisticated upbringing, or by the misrepresentation of consequences," and spelled out some corollary crimes having to do with selling and hiring (Whitfield). Seven years later, in 1968, the Supreme Court of Canada rejected his claim for damages from the employer, on the basis that his contract of employment was entirely clear and "not contrary to public policy."[198]

After moving south with Whitfield, breaking up with him and returning to Great Whale, Witaltuk went to work as an interpreter for the provincial government, and married a federal fishery officer. "We got married in the north, Eskimo style," she told a Canadian Press correspondent in 1969. "You fall in love with a girl and you go to bed with her. I had to bow gracefully out of Terry's life. I was expecting a child. We came down to this civilization of my husband's and we had to get married all over again."[199]

Padlo was wry on the subject of white pontificating, but Witaltuk was downright waspish. "Canadians go around saying: 'There is no discrimination in my country.' They are dreaming. Pure and sweet Canada is neither pure nor sweet."[200]

A year and a half later, the founding meeting of Inuit Tapirisat (Inuit Brotherhood, in English) was convened in Toronto. Mary Panigusiq attended and remarked, "It is all very well that the government sponsor meetings of Inuit on what the government likes, but we Inuit have to meet with our fellow Inuit and make our own plans also" ("Transcript of First ITC Meeting"). Plans to formulate a substantial land claim, for example. The following year there was a pan-Arctic meeting in Pangnirtung. William Tagoona was there as a reporter for *Inuktitut*. Before leaving Ottawa he was warned by other staffers to be careful, as this was to be a political meeting. Recalling the moment in an interview thirty years later he said,

> To us it was almost like a dream to talk about running our own
> affairs, settling land claims – whatever land claims was . . .
> Everything was very new, very strange . . .
>   . . . If you look at the yearbooks of the Churchill
> Vocational Centre, a residential school many Eastern Arctic
> Inuit attended in the 60's and 70's, your question would see
> its answer. After graduating many students had plans to work

as a cashier for the Hudson Bay Company or as a Heavy Equipment Operator. No one talked about one day becoming an Area Manager for the Government, we thought only white people were able to do those kinds of jobs . . .

. . . People like Tagak [Curley] and Charlie [Watt] were giving us the message that the world is there for us to take, that we can dream bigger dreams than the dream given to us at residential schools. To go from wanting to be a cashier to wanting one's own government was quite a big jump. (Tagoona, 10, 12)

2.

The long project of language reform, part of which began at the San, was a Euro-Canadian initiative that the Inuit assimilated, though reluctantly and only partially.

During the lengthy gestation of the land claims agreement that produced Nunavut, the Inuit were also being enrolled in the Canadian nation, that is into the "imagined political community" to use Benedict Anderson's famous phrase, by means of myriad print and photographic representations disseminated in southern Canada, but also into their own shared community by old and new media (Anderson, 5).[201]

Anderson's imagined political community is such that "regardless of the actual inequality and exploitation that may prevail in each, the nation is always conceived as a deep, horizontal comradeship" (7). This comradeship is *imagined*, because personal acquaintance between thousands and millions is impossible; one knows only a few, and imagines the rest. Assisting the imagination during the condensation of nations was "print-capitalism." At first the book, which is "in a rather special sense . . . the first modern-style mass-produced industrial commodity" (34), and then the newspaper, which involves us in "mass ceremony" (35), help the individual to conjure the other members of his or her nation.

Compare Marshall McLuhan, who says, "It may well be that print and nationalism are axiological or co-ordinate, simply because by print a people *sees* itself for the first time. The vernacular in appearing in high visual definition affords a glimpse of social unity co-extensive with vernacular boundaries. And more people have experienced this visual unity of their native tongues *via* the newspaper than through the book" (217).

Media massify. Two more points from Anderson's genetic scheme are relevant here. First, before print can work its magic fusion, standardized print languages must be assembled from the plethora of spoken idiolects, and second, once the product, "nation-ness," a "cultural artefact," has been engendered, it is "'modular,' capable of being transplanted, with varying degrees of self-consciousness, to a great variety of social terrains" (Anderson, 4). The production of this cultural artifact among the newly gathered Inuit communities in Ungava and Baffin circa 1960–1970 by the elaboration of a standardized written language was the project to which, on the initiative of the Canadian government, Raymond Gagné, one-time teacher at the Mountain San, applied himself.

There exists, amid the glorious profusion of the internet, a November 1957 recording of a CBC Television program called *Fighting Words*, in which Gagné figures among the contestants in a conversational game. The object of the show was to identify the author of a quotation, which was then discussed by the panellists. Joining the host, Nathan Cohen, were three other contestants: René Lévesque, then animateur of *Point de mire*; Pierre Trudeau, then editor of *Cité Libre*; and Solange Chaput-Rolland, then editor of *Points de vue*. Gagné was still at the San. The topic of the evening seems to have been something like "Quebec, what and whither?" and the second quotation read was, "No country is enriched by the coexistence of two cultures if one half of the population cannot appropriate the cultural product of the other half." (Canadian historian Hilda Neatby was eventually tagged as the source.) Gagné commented, "I think you can help another culture to benefit from your own by developing yours on a very solid basis and inwardly, from the inside . . . The point I want to make is that if you develop it strong, inwardly, other people will be forced to recognize you" ("Trudeau and Lévesque team up for Fighting Words").

Gagné brought this conviction to his work at the San, where he transformed his task from teacher of English to teacher of Inuktitut – and he seems to have deepened that commitment as he continued his linguistic work, first as a lexicographer and orthographer of the Inuit language for Northern Affairs, and subsequently as a strong advocate of the maintenance of Aboriginal languages at the Université du Québec à Chicoutimi. There he was engaged in a provincial project to "Amerindianize" the schooling of the Inuit, the Montagnais, the Cree and four other indigenous peoples. Underlying the commitment was a sharp sense of peril, arising by analogy from Gagné's perception of Quebec's struggle for cultural survival in the seventies ("French Canada").[202]

Unless the native language becomes the language of instruction, taught by native speakers of it (fully encultured individuals whose behaviour and attitudes are familiar to the children), with English or French taught as second languages, assimilation into the majority culture is inevitable in the long term (Gagné, "The Maintenance of Native Languages").

Following his stint at the San, in 1955 Gagné took a master of arts at the University of Montreal under Gilles Lefebvre. His thesis was "A Phonemic Analysis of an Eastern Hudson Bay Eskimo Dialect with Special Reference to Orthographic Unification," furthering Lefebvre's commission from Northern Affairs to standardize the Inuit spelling – a task dependent on accurately discerning the phonology of the language, which was dependent on sorting through the dialect differences that were complicating matters. This in turn was partly dependent on correcting the mishearing of certain sounds by the European transcribers – French, English and German speakers – who had begun the work of distilling a formalized representation of Inuktitut from the varieties of Inuit speech. To achieve greater objectivity, Gagné used an apparatus called a kymograph, an instrument that recorded variations in sound waves, in his research.

In the Eastern Arctic, converting a sound knowledge of the spoken language into a written form with a standard spelling was more complicated still, as it involved, first of all, the use of two sets of characters, syllabic and alphabetic, and secondly, the dilemma of securing consent to subordinate the dialects to one pan-Arctic written language.

After completing his thesis at Montreal, Gagné went on to the Sorbonne for further studies, and thence to Copenhagen, with the hope of comparing Greenlandic to the Canadian language, in order to align the spelling of each with the other. By 1959 he was able to publish "In Defence of a Standard Phonemic Spelling in Roman Letters for the Canadian Eskimo Language." The following year, working with the linguistics section of the welfare division in Northern Affairs, he began instructing four Inuit in the new system. These individuals were from Fort George (now Chisasibi), Pond Inlet (or Mittimatalik) and Aklavik, and this experience yielded a tentative standard orthograpy. Elijah Erkloo, Alex Spalding and others were recruited to expand the circle to Inuit vocational students at Kingston, among others (Spalding, "'No Frigate Like a Book'").

Spalding had been a Hudson's Bay man at Aivilik (Repulse Bay) where he learned the language under the tutelage of Thomas Kusugaq. The pair published translations of myths and also a dictionary, now available online with other tools. Spalding likened the change from syllabic to alphabetic script to that from twenty-five-cycle to sixty-cycle electric power; in other words, the evolution was inevitable because the latter was technically superior.[203]

When the language reformers took their painstakingly developed gift to the population, it was not accepted. There was indifference and resistance. Inuit chose to emphasize their particularity by retaining the customary form of writing, a script that they had made their own, and the preference was made official in 1976 with the adoption of a dual orthography, the work of an Inuit Language Commission.[204]

As Kenn Harper points out the need was for intra–Eastern Arctic written communication, not a pan-Arctic means of literary enculturation, and the need was satisfied by modifying syllabics

("Inuktitut Writing Systems"). What the Inuit Language Commission ratified was a dual and interchangeable Roman and syllabic orthography. Each syllabic character has a corresponding character or set of characters in the Roman script, so that transliteration is seamless. Syllabics has since been brought forward into digitized word processing and typography as well, and the language itself is adding terms just as the country's Euro-Canadian languages do. In this way, the response to Gagné's government-sponsored proposals, though initially negative, did in the end work toward his ultimate aim, the preservation and maintenance of the language – though this is not yet assured. Nor has standardization of the spoken language been achieved.

The details of all this are complex, but from the perspective of the contribution of print to the "broad horizontal comradeship" that makes for the unity of the nation, reproduction, distribution and their costs are what count. San newsletters were mimeographed – at first hand-lettered, and later typed when syllabic machines were built. This was awkward because the keys had to be hit very hard to cut through the wax coating in order to make a printable stencil. Alootook Ipellie, in reminiscing about his days in the early seventies putting out the newsletter of the Inuit Tapirisat, recalled that the greatest difficulties were inventing Inuit equivalents for English words, and hammering the keys of the "thousand-pound typewriter" that was in use before the "heaven-sent" IBM Selectric arrived (Ipellie). The limiting factor for mimeograph reproduction was the stencil, which would become worn and eventually tear, but the operation of printing itself was fairly fast. For larger quantities, the offset process was possible. Whatever the difficulties, a great many periodicals appeared in the sixties and seventies.[205]

But how much reading and writing actually goes on today? Parallel developments in communication, particularly the spread of Inuktitut language radio, may have made writing and reading redundant as the means to nation-ness. In addition, radio and television have exposed the young to dialects other than that of their own region, so that mutual comprehension is becoming easier. It seems probable that the main means of producing the Inuit public was not print but radio; and what is the standing of text in the current mix of radio, television, telephone and internet, the last of which fuses all media and serves equally well the passive many and the active few?

The question of standardization came to the fore again when certain obligations were embedded in 2008's Inuit Language Protection Act. The act and its companion, the Official Languages Act, were written in response to the prevalence of English in the public space. This legislation seems to give the government of Nunavut authority to do what Ottawa could not: impose a dialect and an orthography, although it is not likely that this authority will come to a test anytime soon.[206]

As the insistence on consensus in matters of language reform has thus far produced mostly sectarianism, it seems likely that not government policy but other influences will determine the outcome for Inuktitut in the Canadian Arctic. Given the intense competition for the attention of each and every Inuk, immersed as they are in the same technical unity of communication as almost all other Canadians and Europeans, what can be the comparative effect of policy, no matter how thoroughly enforced?

The last word goes to Jay Arnakak, a translator and former civil servant on the front lines of the struggle for Inuktitut. On his blog, *Qituttugaujara*, in the fall of 2011, Arnakak said that "language is a social phenomenon, where the narrative is key to capturing and engaging the student." However, he continued, story is absent from Inuktitut instruction because Inuit myths and legends are regarded as religious and so tacitly excluded from school, and there are no pedagogically trained elders to tell stories and demonstrate proper grammar, so students are just memorizing vocabulary. Moreover, the loyalty to syllabics is self-defeating; use of standard Roman orthography would ease reading and make the building blocks of the language more evident to the student. Arnakak sums up with this:

> Developing linguistic competence and language acquisition do not require high-tech gizmos and gadgets nor even money and funding that will never be given in sufficient amounts; only our engagement and participation in the social phenomenon

197

called language as human to human can we make the difference. The Inuit narrative has so much to offer, especially when we reflect upon not just our long-long history as an Arctic people but also as contemporary society working it out through recent colonialist past and all the teachable moments inherent in that experience. In telling our story do possibilities become real objects of contemplation and imagination.

3.

Inuit returning from southern Canada after an absence of one or two or three years, with some or no disability, with old skills dulled and/or new skills acquired, came back to a world often changing more rapidly than the one they had left, especially after 1960 when camp life was being curtailed. In the earliest days they resumed the previous life – man, woman or child – with no preparation; later returnees might pause at a rehab centre.

Ebba Olofsson, a Swedish (now Canadian) researcher of what she calls narrative identity (after Paul Ricoeur) has interviewed TB evacuees and found that some had difficulty going back on the land and sleeping in impermanent shelters because they still felt the effects of surgery or were somewhat enfeebled by the disease. Some were also uneasy because the emphasis on hygiene in the hospitals had made a lasting impression. They were reluctant to share cups and worried about the state of their blankets. One of Olofsson's informants said he had become accustomed to regular mealtimes, and was made anxious by the lack of routine when he rejoined his family.

A 1962 radio talk prepared by social worker Phyllis Harrison told the story of a "fairly typical" couple undergoing trial by TB around 1960. Kelough and Anarwakoloo, parents of four, lived three days from Iqaluit. Kelough became ill and went out to Hamilton after Northern Affairs agreed to foster-home payments to help her sister care for the children. Before her return, her doctor wrote Harrison advising that Kelough was not strong enough to go back on the land. She would have to make a different life for herself. Her husband was referred to the rehab centre, whose functionaries placed him in a job, and provided temporary housing when Kelough arrived (Harrison).

The great ingathering that was underway was often experienced, quite analogously to the medical evacuations, as captivity. Seasonal travel between campsites that had been used for generations was greatly reduced. The experience in the Baffin region, as recounted by witnesses to the Qikiqtani Truth Commission, was a Canadian policy of resettlement carried through with no coordinated, considered strategy. In some cases people who went into town expecting to return to their camp left their belongings behind, only to have their sod house destroyed by a bulldozer. Concentrating teams of idle, hungry sled dogs together with large numbers of people was not workable. Ordinances were proclaimed obliging owners to tie their dogs, but explanations were scanty and consultation with Inuit did not occur. Rope was ineffectual to hold strong-jawed dogs, and chain was expensive. It was not only free-roving animals that were destroyed; dogs were shot outside trading posts while their owner was doing business inside. When dogs were shot, usually by the RCMP, the owner was left stranded in town, unable to travel or hunt, resulting in grief for the lost animals, homesickness, hunger and poverty for the family. Some men were able to replace their teams with skidoos or other dogs, but many could not. Moreover, the snow machines were not as reliable as dogs, and gas and repairs were costly. Housing rents, which the Inuit believed to be fixed, were raised over time ("QTC Background Reports: Updates & Executive Summaries"). In short, resettlement in Baffin was carried out to meet the goals of the Ottawa administrators, with no apparent consideration of the immediate implications on the day-to-day needs of the Inuit.

People went, over ten or fifteen years, from a semi-nomadic life on the land, searching out the food animals or travelling to an annual rendezvous with them, to a less physically strenuous town life; from isolation to sustained telecommunications and air service (not very frequent at first); and from episodic scarcity to continuous low-grade,

199

very expensive abundance, supplemented with a portion of country food. The young became more numerous, and some of the settlements became busy with the Euro-Canadian style of business. In 1950 there were thought to be about seven hundred camps. By 1970, these people had mostly come together to reside much of the year in only forty settlements (Bruemmer, 143). Each of these communities grew at its own rate and in a different manner, and the greatest part of the movement into them occurred after 1960.[207]

Through all the changes, tuberculosis continued, if not to thrive, certainly to enjoy a modest career and evade the various poisons. In March 1962, at the moment of the San's transition from sanatorium to outpatient or domiciliary treatment centre, the leading Ontario practitioners were assembled to discuss the change. Invited to comment on the question of future TB research, they said that three things were required: first, something better than the tuberculin test was needed to help in case finding; second, a better anti-microbial agent; and third, a better immunizing agent. They did not like it that BCG blurred the tuberculin test, and they were uncertain about what might in fact be the best practice with BCG. As to how to obtain that better vaccine, there was sharp disagreement. Woolf, from the cardiopulmonary lab at Toronto General, thought a crash program "might develop as it did in several of the wartime programs where a great deal of energy, research and money were used to reach a solution of a pressing problem."[208] Riley Armstrong, who had run the labs at Mountain for many years, thought not. It was a "misconception" that if there was a "practical problem" you could solve it by spending money. Historically, "the practical things that have come out of research have really popped up as sort of offshoots from much bigger cases of research."[209] Wicks, from Weston, was worried, as were the rest, about the growing public complacency, and the perception that TB was controlled.

Some months later, in August 1962, the three hundred twenty-nine Inuit and sixteen Euro-Canadians from Arviat (now in Nunavut) were given chest x-rays and the TB cases were flown out. The community then had an epidemic of mumps, another of measles and a third of rubella, a disease innocuous for the most part but sometimes causing deafness or cataracts in the unborn if contracted by the mother. In January 1963, a second set of x-rays turned up eighty cases of TB. So much for control.

Around 1960 it was learned that Inuit are rapid metabolizers of INH compared to Euro-Canadians. (About sixty percent of other Aboriginals share this characteristic with the northerners.) Since the effectiveness of the drug is proportional to the amount present in the blood and the length of time it remains there intact, changes in these two variables can affect the course of treatment. When an INH-streptomycin combination is given daily, the difference between slow and rapid metabolizers is inconsequential.[210] However, doctors mistrustful of self-administration in domiciliary programs decided that directly supervised treatment once a week would be safer. With such a long interval between doses, the rate at which the drug was broken down began to matter. Simply raising the dose was not possible because of the drug's toxicity. In the seventies therefore clinicians began compounding INH with a matrix that slowed its release into the bloodstream. This allowed them to triple the dose without triggering side effects (Jeanes, Schaefer and Eidus, 483–87).

Not only active, but inactive and even merely infected cases were being treated – *chemoprophylaxis* is the term – in an effort to mop up. In 1976, S. Grzybowski, K. Styblo and E. Dorken published a fifteen-year overview (1960–1975) of "Tuberculosis in Eskimos." This dealt with Greenland and Alaska, as well as the Canadian North. According to these researchers, "The Eskimos are co-operative in taking anti-tuberculosis drugs. The best evidence is that there was, during the entire fifteen-year period under study, only one chronic tuberculosis excretor among the 851 bacillary cases (including relapses) discovered and treated at that time" (Grzybowski, Styblo and Dorken, S38). This does not quite square with the assertion of Jeanes, Schaefer and Eidus from 1973, that there was "frequent patient delinquency in adhering to the recommended treatment regiment due to poor social conditions, frustration, alcoholism and lack of proper communication" (484). What this contradiction seems to mean is that treatment persisted past failures, which were all detected.

The disease persisted but declined in incidence (though not to all-Canada levels) until the nineties, when it began to creep up again. Darkening the prospect was the increase in diabetes, which, like HIV, lowers resistance to TB by hampering elements of the immune response. The diabetic are at least three times likelier to develop active disease. In 2003, physician and novelist Kevin Patterson, writing about his experience with what he calls the patient predator, described the situation of one of his Inuit patients, a twenty-seven-year-old woman living in Arviat. She had a large cavity in one lung, did not respond to treatment, went south, did not get better and was sent back home at her own insistence. It might as well have been 1945, and for her particular strain of the bug, apparently it was. "She is suspicious of doctors and nurses and takes medication only episodically" (Patterson, "TB"). But episodically would not quite do.

Mycobacterium tuberculosis, held in check in Canada, meanwhile thrives in other parts of the world,[211] and the search for better antimicrobials and better combinations of them continues. In early 2014 the World Health Organization believed that there were five so-called first-line drugs[212] and a further eight second-line choices. The first-line drugs are preferred for their low toxicity and strong action by comparison with the fallback substances. Isoniazid remains the single most effective. Streptomycin has been replaced by rifampin in two-drug regimes, and PAS has dropped to the second-line. Since the mechanism by which strains resistant to this or that drug become dominant in the bacillary population under drug pressure is understood, the problem of control is more than ever one of ensuring that treatment is thorough: the right drug on the least onerous schedule for the patient, both in terms of time needed to complete and side effects to be endured.

As for immunization, BCG remains the only vaccine in wide use. In 2006, for example, seventy percent of previously unvaccinated Afghani children received BCG and polio shots (Graeme Smith, "Troops' Goals Appear More Distant"). However, knowledge of the organism itself has improved and with it the hope of new vaccines. We know how the various antibiotics interfere with the metabolism of the bacillus. The genetic code of several strains of TB is also known, so that, technically, we may be nearing the end of our struggle with this microbe. Technically.

However, as our experience and understanding of the disease and its agent has grown, so has our appreciation of the recalcitrance of the political situation. Grzybowski, Styblo and Dorken closed their survey on an optimistic note. The decline of TB among Inuit over a decade or so was much the same as had occurred in the "developed countries over the past 50–100 years" (S42) and for the same reason. The incidence of disease was down because the risk of exposure was down. However, in the developed countries this was brought about very gradually by "rising economic standards rather than by specific anti-tuberculosis measures" (S42). Those measures, initially, were costly, as hospitalization was involved. (And direct means, in themselves, have not been quite enough to do what is needed.) Nonetheless, the doctors concluded, costs need not be an obstacle for others: "The basic diagnostic and treatment programs which were the backbone of the success in Eskimos could also be effective to a lesser degree in countries with limited financial resources. Sputum bacteriology can be substituted for chest X-rays and thorough and appropriate chemotherapy can be given on an out-patient basis. It is possible to reduce tuberculosis rates rapidly if the following principles are implemented – each infectious case must be diagnosed promptly and each diagnosed case must be cured" (S42–3).

This has so far proven politically difficult in large parts of the world. It seems that we must either have something as effective as the polio vaccine (whose delivery also entails political problems but of a more manageable nature), or return to the resignation of the nineteenth century. But remaining in our part of the world, are we in fact able to find and cure every single case in the Arctic before they infect others?

For a year and a half ending in June 1999 a Danish woman named Helle Møeller worked as a TB nurse in three Nunavut communities. She found that some patients interrupted their course of treatment, and that some treatment went unsupervised because the patient did not report as requested. The absolute numbers are small, but so is the population – about thirty thousand – making the rates much higher. Switching to anthropology, Møeller set out to learn why, and came up with answers and recommendations that she offered in a thesis for the University of Copenhagen. She drew on Foucault for her theoretical framework:

> I believe that the development in Europe from a sovereign power over life and death to a normalizing and medicalizing power invested in life is mirrored by the development that took place during a much shorter time-span in the Canadian Arctic. Before the Canadian government had realised the possibilities of the Arctic, its inhabitants were allowed to die as a consequence of contact with explorers, traders and missionaries. Once the value of the Arctic was recognised, and in its attempt to gain sovereignty, the Canadian government also attempted to manage and normalise its Inuit inhabitants, in order to have healthy bodies living in the north. The relocations and medicalization described above did this, and I believe this normalization, in the form of continuing colonization and acculturation, is ongoing. (54–55)[213]

Møeller emphasizes three points that arise directly from her work as a tuberculosis nurse, and from inquiries she made in an effort to determine why her TB work kept hitting snags. One is the observation that chaotic living day to day makes it hard to keep to a therapeutic course. Another has to do with the rude, resentful and therefore self-defeating attitudes of some health-care providers. The third is about the persisting Inuit perspective on wellness, and the persistent deprecation of that perspective by Euro-Canadian medical personnel.

Møeller interviewed thirty-six people, including a number of "Qallunaat health professionals" (58), in Iqaluit and another, unnamed community not far from the capital. Many of the women with whom she spoke told of being threatened, sexually abused and beaten. They also told of men whom they knew to have been abused by a Euro-Canadian teacher, and of one who "was sent to boarding school where priests sexually abused him" (71). She talked to a couple of deeply unhappy young women who had been dealt a very bad hand. One came from a family whose parents separated while she was in her teens. She moved in with her father, a Euro-Canadian. He used drugs, and would take some of the money the daughter earned, money that she needed to buy food for the younger children. When she began to refuse him, he asked her to leave, which she did. Her brothers now have problems with drugs and alcohol.

The other interviewee, who had been treated for TB, had difficulty in following the prescribed course because of the situation in her home. Her parents spent their money on alcohol, and did not put food in the house. Taking medications without eating upset her stomach. Because her parents did not support her treatment, and because she could not always be found to be given her medicine, she was taken into custody and kept in the hospital. However, she said, "*I used to sneak out and go home, find my sister and brother alone, my parents gone out drinking . . . I was isolated for two weeks and I worried about my brother and sister. I had to sneak out. I didn't want my sister and brother to be alone while my parents were drinking*" (italics original; Møeller, 72).[214]

Subsequently the woman's father died. The mother took a new partner, but while he himself worked, he bought drugs and did not want the mother to work, so food was likely in short supply again. The mother was passive and weepy, and the daughter had to take charge of the other children. She did not go to school because she could not get up early enough, though she would have liked to attend and wanted to become a teacher.

Møeller remarks that this woman's "life circumstances are too overwhelming to allow for good health and in my interpretation too overwhelming to allow for attending school regularly. She blamed herself, however, for not attending school and for the lack of ability to adhere to her treatment for TB. I see [this woman] as someone who has internalized the rules of the *disciplines*, (Foucault, 1991, 1995) in the form of the healthcare system and the educational system" (73).

Møeller finds resentment (she calls it "blaming the victims" [78]) and even bullying among health-care workers who are vexed by the unruliness of the clientele, and was told that doctors and nurses were aloof and withholding. The patient was not given explanations. One woman, suspected of having reactivated TB and given drugs that caused severe side effects, was then discharged without being told that she was now negative, nor that she had been tuberculous in the first place. (How she learned this in the absence of communication from the medical staff is not indicated.) One young woman who avoided her meds because they made her dizzy and nauseous reported being told by a nurse that *"we're just going to let you stop and if you get sick it's going to be your own fault. If the TB comes back to you and gets worse we're not going to do anything about it"* (italics original; quoted in Møeller, 65).

As Møeller herself remarks, none of this bad feeling is unique to the North, but can and does happen everywhere. The deeper problem is that Inuit have a view on these matters that is discounted. Møeller thinks that Euro-Canadian comportment could be better. Visiting medical personnel could learn and show respect for the Inuit perception of the patterning of health and sickness, not only in their dealings with patients and their families, but also with their students. This would generally improve morale and so serve indirectly to alleviate other problems, born of anger and resentment, that make it difficult to look after one's health. Beyond that, she wants stability of medical personnel and Inuitization of health services. The second seems attainable, but the first is unlikely. Neither a Euro-Canadian nor an Inuk physician or nurse is likely to choose to spend most of their time in a northern practice rather than commuting from Montreal.

Euro-Canadian incomprehension and indifference to Inuit medical views is an old and persisting problem. George Wenzel published the same grievance in 1981:

In two instances within my experience at Clyde River, one an accidental death and the other a severe epileptic-like event, root causes were sought and found by the Inuit not in the completely plausible explanations of Western medicine, but in social environmental relations of those individuals earlier in their lives . . . For Inuit, treatment and prognosis rest heavily on the etiological background, both physical and non-physical, of the patient's complaint. If causation may be related to a serious spiritual/psycho-social event or action, the treatment must be adjusted to the cause. (11)

He cites the example of an elderly hunter who developed a rash and complications that prevented him from hunting. Neither the staff at the local nursing station nor in Montreal, where he went for several months, could help. However, an Inuk from a neighbouring camp remembered that in the past the man had not properly disposed of a caribou carcass. Perhaps there was a connection with the rash. The hunter, reminded of his past omission, agreed, and shortly the rash faded. The point is that others, not only the (invariably Euro-Canadian) health-care providers, have a role to play in diagnosis and treatment: "Inuit today are faced squarely by a dichotomy: an effective system on the Western pattern focused on physical causation; or an approach which is holistic vis-à-vis Inuit normative associations, but which the Western model views as anachronistic, or at least unscientific/unmanageable" (Wenzel, 13). In this circumstance, Inuit felt that the medical services on offer were technically good, but "saw themselves as being gradually alienated from a set of responsibilities that was theirs as Inuit" (ibid., 13).

But there is another, more disturbing recurrence. The engineers of the TB control program on the Navajo reservation came to see that when technology was transferred between societies, both need to change. Having put a good deal of effort into fostering change in the receiving society, the organizers realized, much too late, that the donor society also needed to change in order to accommodate the new way of delivering care, or else it would not be perpetuated. All would have been in vain. What Møeller reported fifty years after intensive delivery of medical services into the Eastern Arctic began suggests that the growing ease of travel had allowed medical personnel to avoid change in the donor society – to transfer medical technique without themselves changing; nor apparently, were the Inuit able to shape the medical art to their own particularities and preferences. One has the impression that some necessary accommodation was not being made – collaboration was not taking place. Obviously it would require extensive study to verify if this is so, and what may be missing, and of course it is impossible for medicine to compensate for every deficiency in nutrition, shelter and satisfaction. It seems equally obvious that respect for tradition and its bearers is by and large worth inculcating as part of the health-care discipline – at least where it will enhance the security and well-being, and therefore the freedom, of each. By and large, because some traditions are not mutually compatible on any basis – although the converse also is true: wherever compatible traditions meet, preservation of both will likely occur.

But collaboration may be growing. Following Møeller's tour of duty, the first decade of the new century saw an alarming increase in TB cases (Zarate). One response has been the organization of Taima TB, a campaign of publicity followed by door-to-door canvassing in Iqaluit by a team of champions, reminiscent of the health visitor program employed on the Navajo reserve for five years or so after 1955 (George).

I have drawn on Patterson and Møeller because they are medical practitioners who have provided first-hand accounts of their experience in the North fifty years on from the period we have been examining. Møeller is a Dane who went to Nunavut as a TB nurse in 1997 and returned in 1999 as an anthropologist in training. Her sample was small but her thesis conveyed the emotional texture of medicalized life. Patterson is a physician and novelist who has worked in the Arctic and the South Pacific, as well as in Afghanistan, and has drawn on his experiences in the first two places in writing *Consumption*, a novel whose punning title connotes the specific disease and the general malaise that comes with excessive indulgence in abundance.

When I am reading Møeller and Patterson however I feel that we have seen them before, the decolonizing crusader, the far-travelling adventurer . . . If we screw up our eyes and squint a little, this pair seems familiar, like Houston and Mowat, or like Johanna van der Woerd who came from Holland with a missionary bent. An old pattern reappears in the new fabric, and the land of extremes remains a lure and a place of discovery and self-making for outsiders.[215]

Some problems have no solution, and of course it is a problem to know which ones they are. But we can learn this only by trying. And then, some solutions prove partial or illusory. So far, directly observed chemotherapy has enabled us to contain, but not eradicate, TB in this country. In the area once served by the Mountain San, about twenty cases a year are detected among a population of half a million. In Nunavut in 2010, the number of new cases reached a ten-year high of one hundred two. The total population was about thirty-three thousand. Most infections were in Iqaluit and Cape Dorset. It would seem then that we must obtain a vaccine, or reconcile ourselves to living with a danger that at some point we may no longer be able to contain. Or, of course, eliminate the chronic poverty and consequent housing deficiencies, bad food and emotional turmoil that nurture the disease – but this is just what we don't seem able to do.

SIX: CONCLUDING REMARKS

1.

Knowledge is power, but if it is to augment the political power, it must be exercised over physical and social distance, and in the case of medical knowledge, the skills, drugs and instruments arising from new knowledge must be sent into all parts of the territory. England was able to grasp Hudson Bay by means of the Hudson's Bay Company and the company's Aboriginal trading partners, who attended at a string of seaboard posts. It was largely by piggybacking on those long supply lines that, after the cession of Rupert's Land (1870) and then the Arctic Archipelago (1880, 1895) to the new entity, Canadian statesmen were able to reach across the distance between the capital and the people over whose land they wished to become sovereign – a wish that the Canadian state itself lacked means to realize.[216] Pending the necessary technological developments, and the accumulation of the wealth to pay for them, an annual shipborne Arctic patrol was the state's instrument to inventory its putative domain and assert its right. Up to 1950 this patrol was conducted mainly from chartered vessels. (The exception was the *Arctic*, originally built for a German Antarctic expedition and purchased by the Canadian government in 1904.) Gradually, assisted by the enlargement of the state's capacities during the European and Pacific wars, the lineaments of power became equal to the pretensions of the politicians. The capacity to build true icebreakers, the proliferation of aircraft of all sizes, including the long-sought helicopter, and the advent of satellite or microwave relay towers to assist communications allowed the dream to become practicable; the decision of the American rulers to maintain the centrality of military spending in the US economy forced it to be realized. A very wild ride ensued. The logic of territorial competition and technological change entailed first the rapid completion of the Canadian colonization of the Arctic, and then almost immediately, like a wound spring uncoiling, the nominal reassignment of authority to its rightful holders and the relinquishing of the undeclared colony to its proper owners, all within a single generation.

In 1854 Laurence Oliphant, the superintendent of Indian Affairs, enunciated the first principle of Canadian-Aboriginal relations as well as anyone has. Reporting on his difficulties in the Saugeen peninsula of Ontario, Oliphant wrote that "so keen was the struggle for land that a surrender of the territory for purpose of sale appeared the only method by which the property of these tribes could be conserved to them. It therefore became an obligation upon the Indian Department to spare no pains in endeavouring to *wring from those whom it protects*, some assent, however reluctant, to the adoption of the only means by which this object could be achieved" (italics original; quoted in Schmalz, 141).

Thirty-five years later, that struggle between Aboriginal and white farmers had extended to the 52nd parallel of the Northwest Territories. The following gives a sense of the relentlessness of the barrage under which Aboriginal economic prospects wilted. This is one of a hundred thousand blows:

> In the summer and fall of 1889 hay was particularly scarce because of drought, frost, and fires that burned large stretches of hay land. It was also in short supply because for weeks at a time the Indians and white settlers had been busy fighting fires and could not attend to haying. In September P.J. Williams, the Battleford Indian agent, urged Commissioner Reed to take steps to set aside at once hay lands that had come to the notice of the settlers, as "nearly everyone who has stock is after these lands." If the land was not secured, there was no alternative but to decrease stock on the reserve. E. Brokowsi of the Dominion Lands office, however, did not

believe such a large additional area was required, particularly in view of the "evident dissatisfaction of white settlers" for whom cattle had become a main source of revenue because of crop failure. The Department of Indian Affairs agreed to abandon claim to 2,080 acres of hay land, and Hayter Reed [deputy superintendent general of Indian Affairs] informed settlers that as he was "desirous to consider the feelings of the settlers as far as possible," he was endeavouring to dispense with a further 1,600 acres. (Carter, 186–87)

Until 1950 or so the Inuit were spared the worst of the aggressions visited upon their more southerly cousins. They had their presumed irreligion corrected, and otherwise were ignored, imposed upon or assisted in about the same measure as southern-dwelling Euro-Canadians, who were not pampered. The exception was access to health services, which was scant, and the burden of disease was high.

Doctors MacCarthy and Laidlaw, who were on the *Nascopie* in 1945, found that food poisoning was common in the summer. In July, eight died at Lake Harbour of something the doctors thought might be botulism. On examining one hundred forty-five people at six ports of call, they found fifteen cases of TB and suspected more. They found also thirty-three cases of eye trouble, mostly conjunctivitis, but also six cases of cataracts and four of corneal ulcer. Also sixteen cases of otitis media, and twenty cases of bronchitis, plus epilepsy, hernia and rheumatism. Scabies. Impetigo. Gastroenteritis. *Et j'en passe.*[217] There were other problems. Ship fever was known to break out in the aftermath of their visit at each port. And the diet was worsening. "For some years past those natives who have been able to establish a good line of credit at a trading post have been supplying themselves with 'white man's food' – so abundantly in some instances as to endanger health. It is held by some authorities that white flour products are definitely harmful, as also are sugar (which is not rationed) and such things as rich jams and honey. Tea has become the favourite drink and like tobacco, is used in quantity whenever it can be obtained."[218]

R. C. Hastings, medical officer on the *N.B. McLean* in 1946, found that during the year previous to his visit, thirteen children were born in the vicinity of Ivujivik on the high eastern shore of Hudson Bay. One was still living.[219] Around the headland, on the Ungava Bay side, a measles epidemic in 1952 killed eleven adults in the region now centred on Quaqtaq – ten percent of the population (Dorais, 28). Gérard Duhaime, in a detailed analysis of thirteen Nunavik villages, found a pronounced gap in the birth rate for the years 1939 to 1948, and especially the five years from 1939 to 1943 – a gap so serious that births were probably below the replacement rate. From 1944 to 1951, the growth rate was almost flat: three-tenths of a percent. After 1955, births increased sharply, and the birth rate continued to increase until after 1970.

In general, it was policy, or rather it was attitude seeking confirmation as policy, to encourage Inuit independence from outside supports. This was somewhat contradictory to the simultaneous project of integrating Inuit hunters into the international economy as trappers or de facto employees of the Hudson's Bay Company. Because trapping was time-consuming and energy-intensive (travel was by dog team and they had to be fed), and because the fox harvest was cyclic, trappers had to be pensioned somehow to get them through the lean times. But then their patrons risked, in their own view, making them dependent on initiative-curbing handouts. The (unexpressed) ideal was to do with the Inuit as had been done historically with the Euro-Canadian poor and make of them indentured servants, company debtors or co-adventurers in the Newfoundland style, that is to say, serfs rather than wards. But then the fur trade failed altogether, and Inuit artistic production came to share the part in North–South commerce once held exclusively by trapping. The co-op set up had the pensioning effect. When wage labour was not available, carving permitted hunting to continue.

After 1940 the firebombing of England, Germany and Japan shifted strategy away from inter-military combat toward the killing of civilians, and this moved another frontier deep into the Arctic. The region began to fill up with visiting southerners and their material, many of them citizens of the United States. In this era of the long-range bomber and the Distant Early Warning line, the Canadian government rediscovered the utility of Her Majesty's Indian Allies. Aboriginals had fought for British North America in the 1770s and on many subsequent occasions, and could now serve again to counter US encroachment in the North.[220]

When the Committee on Eskimo Affairs began meeting in the fall of 1952, it revived a predecessor, now named the Advisory Committee on Northern Development, to act as its conduit to cabinet. It did so, according to R. Quinn Duffy, because "the cabinet wanted to be informed of all activities in the Arctic, to have periodic reports of proposed developments, to receive recommendations of what could be done to promote Canadian initiative and to have Canada take the lead rather than let the United States set the pace in areas of Joint Participation" (149).

As had been the custom already for more than a century, the jealous keepers of Canadian sovereignty responded to the perceived American challenge with a program of defensive expansion organized and financed largely by the state.[221] After 1945 the Canadian state possessed technical means adequate (almost) to the task of projecting its interests in the northern territories to counter the Americans, and hired and organized its own servants to displace the incumbents. The Dominion built an apparatus to mediate between the churches, the HBC and the police, and eventually to supersede them in many functions. This apparatus had two principal branches: Health and Welfare's northern divisions and the Department of Northern Affairs and Natural Resources, those resources being its primary raison d'être.

Of course, if occupation and use were the criteria, then the logical rivals for sovereignty in the North were not the Americans or the Danes, but the Inuit themselves – and so it has come to pass. But in 1950 there was no Inuit polity to make the claim, nor was anyone soliciting their opinions in the matter. This problem would go away if the Inuit were mere Canadians; but what if they were the equivalent of other First Nations peoples, and therefore wards of the state? In fact, this question had been answered by the Supreme Court of Canada in 1935 in the affirmative. (The point was argued between Ottawa and Quebec, with no representation from the Inuit.) However, because

Aboriginal policy was seen to have been a financial failure, not to be repeated if it could be avoided, those concerned with northern affairs went on ignoring the implications and affected to consider Inuit of all regions as ordinary Canadian citizens. (There was also the slight matter of Aboriginal title, best left in abeyance as long as possible, or preferably ignored altogether.)

In any case, developments both technical and political were making the difference of no *immediate* practical importance, because southern Canadians were themselves becoming wards of the state. Depression and war and great discontent had led the rulers – their capacity much increased by a centralized tax power and a greatly expanded bureaucracy (from 46,000 functionaries in 1939 to 116,000 in 1945) – to offer services previously considered profligate if not corrupting. The feasibility of old-age security, unemployment insurance and a degree of socialized medicine decided, the economic question then reduced to the costs of delivery. These were higher in the territories and Newfoundland. And this fact, among others, made evacuation preferable to in-country treatment for the organizers.

Once the state took responsibility for the welfare of people in all regions equally, administrators had to acknowledge and deal with the burden of tuberculosis in the North. The upshot was that the sanatoria, like residential schools, gained "entire possession" of the tuberculous Inuit – not only of the children, but of all the tuberculous; and not only of the tuberculous, but of all Inuit. Under the regime installed to combat the epidemic, the entire population was essentially at the disposal of a team of medical examiners, who made a circuit of Hudson Bay and Baffin once a year on the *C. D. Howe*. In 1950, this population numbered about ten thousand; a seventh part of these eventually came south for a stay of a year or more. Beginning in 1954 Inuit from the Eastern Arctic went to Hamilton, and in 1955 and '56, there were about two hundred seventy there at any one time, after which the numbers tapered off rapidly through 1962.[222] In 1981, the census recorded twenty-three thousand Inuit (Grygier, 85). This was power unprecedented in the North, amplified by new technologies and exercised without impediment from politically unorganized and physically debilitated Inuit families and groups, who were fearful, deprived of their dietary mainstays by the usurpations or poor advice of outsiders and reduced in numbers by many earlier incidents of disease.

The medical evacuations were an extreme of colonial assertion and Aboriginal subordination not previously seen in the North, although matched also by a number of relocation experiments occurring at the same time (Tester and Kulchyski).

The decisions to conduct mass surveys and evacuate the infected, just when southern sanatoria needed patients for their emptying beds, was resisted by many, and not only Inuit. (It bears repeating that the evacuation policy was decided in advance of the chemotherapeutic revolution that emptied those beds.) Willis, who organized it, and Phillips, who oversaw it as one part of a comprehensive seizure of authority by Northern Affairs, believed it was an obligation of the department to, in Oliphant's phrase, "*wring from those whom it protects, some assent*" to evacuation and treatment (italics original; quoted in Schmalz, 141). But there was an immense difference between the two operations – the reduction of tuberculosis in the Arctic, unlike the dispossession of the people of the Saugeen and many others, was of benefit to the Inuit. Euro-Canadians were sharing long-sought and hard-earned knowledge – but this sharing was and continues to be limited. As Wenzel and Møeller report, the delivery of medical benefits has not been altered by Inuit as other Euro-Canadian forms have been and there has been dissatisfaction with this rigidity. The resettlement policy, carried through in part in order to improve access to medical services, inadvertently produced the living conditions that have allowed TB to persist and even flourish. The lesson seems to be that only a specific against the bacillus, or a vaccine, can defeat it. Despite many successes, we have begun to lose ground here in Canada and almost everywhere, because other approaches have been beyond our powers. We have been politically incapable of removing the general conditions that nurture the agents of infectious disease in large parts of the world. In particular, Canadians have been unable or unwilling to improve those conditions in northern and rural areas. This is not a technical problem.

In determining what was "best for the Eskimo," all concur that relieving them of incapacitating and life-threatening disease was obviously for the best. Beyond that, the answer would depend on how much of Inuit particularity would be going forward into the future. But then, in what did that particularity consist, exactly? And who is asking? That is, who did the Euro-Canadians think that they themselves were? In 1850, most of the active fraction of whites thought that they were members of a superior, but thankfully beneficent, race, charged by the Creator with the task of uplifting the inferior peoples – or, if that were impossible, at least with supervising them in order that they too would contribute to the right ordering of the world (and, of course, to its work). Most thought this, but not all; there has always been vocal and energetic minority opinion. By 1950, the sense of superiority remained, but the racism, that is, the ideology of race hierarchy that distinguishes articulate racism from formless bigotry, was dissipated, and replaced with a kind of Darwinist progressivism. Whites now understood themselves as not only the benefactors and disciplinarians, but also inadvertent destroyers. This was owing to a fatal entanglement of both whites and Aboriginals in a forced march of progress through nature, with squalor and disease for by-products.

The provision of medical services to the North, and the extension of other entitlements of the welfare state (the right to revenue, as C. B. Macpherson calls it) provided the moral basis for Canada's presumptive authority in the region. But underneath the question of what was best for the Inuit always ran another: By what right was Canada deciding what was best? Once Health and Welfare had shrunk the TB threat and Northern Affairs had resolved the dispersion-concentration debate in favour of concentration, the government's work expanded still further, and the question of right came forward strongly and was insisted upon.

Again and again the histories of the period dip into the extensive archival record to retrieve expressions of ambiguity. The experience of colonialists is frequently one of frustration and futility. The way out is finally to accept defeat, admit ignorance and enter into genuine collaboration to realize the ecumenical ambition implicit in the missionary stance – implicit but usually buried and walled over. But true respect is risky because it accepts the possibility of conversion to the other's perspective. Moreover, it is fundamentally inarguable. The mark of respect is to accept where one cannot agree, and to set aside the question or the thing in dispute. Respect entails renunciation. But what is a missionary without a mission? What is a nation without a vocation?

In the words of Robert Paine, in 1977,

> ambiguity in a colonial situation is especially likely to occur where there is an awareness by one or both sides of their involvement in the maintenance of the other's illegitimate position . . . Colonizers [whites] have become increasingly aware of how they devaluate the colonized, the Inuit. Now this tends to produce among the whites themselves a sense of self devaluation, ushering in one of the paradoxes of welfare colonialism in the North: as the whites become more aware that "colonial" behaviour is in conflict with . . . egalitarian philosophy, so their position becomes presented to them as one in which the more they succeed, the more they fail. What of the Inuit? Here it may be a case of the weak finding some measure of protecting [sic] through the confusion of the strong, and one asks what else, besides Inuit-white misunderstandings and the ambiguities that whites suffer among themselves, stands between the Inuit and their ethnocide? (28)

Whites and Inuit entered a time of serious *prise de conscience* with regard to one another, from which the Inuit emerged possessed of a political self-consciousness that eventually found expression in Nunavut and Nunavik. Whites came out divided, many with a drastically revised judgement on the past. This was now seen as a long failure to deal equitably with Aboriginals, a failure due to white pride, ignorance and covetousness. The *Eskimo consciousness* of southerners had to be expanded if the North was to be added into Canada – the self-conception of Canadians would have to be elaborated to include that region and its peoples; that is, symbolic integration would have to occur, and did occur.

Defensive expansion, usually termed conquest by those who find themselves in the way of it, had been resisted by un-British North Americans in the not-yet-Canadian West. These local solidarities were broken by force or weakened by treaty and pushed aside, but failed to evaporate as the founders hoped; rather a long war of attrition ensued and continues to this moment. By 1950 it was clear to most that Canadian aggressions must cease, but few Euro-Canadians were ready to draw the lesson of Quebec – that the security, and therefore allegiance, of peoples existing before and persisting within Confederation could only be assured on the basis of guarantees for homeland and language. While medical professionals and administrators struggled with various aspects of an *Eskimo problem* that they judged was theirs to address, they did so amid a slow-growing Inuit sense that in fact the problem was rather their own. The Inuit did not wish to surrender all particularity, but neither could they hold to or revert to tradition, and in any case the preservation of tradition itself requires innovation and adaptation as circumstances change. Once this was understood and accepted by both Inuit and their Euro-Canadian supervisors, the latter had to negotiate the emergence of a political form for Inuit particularity, and this occurred and is being continuously modified, just as the forms of the larger Canadian polity are continuously modified.

Regarded under its philosophical aspect, the *Eskimo problem*, like that of cultural persistence generally, is that of rational pluralism. In its bare logical expression, the problem is that of achieving a unity – in this case, that of the Canadian nation – that does not obviate the parts that are to be unified, since otherwise there is nothing to unite. It follows that the parts, to be discernible as parts, must themselves have a unity and it is this last, the integrity of the parts – including the preference of those whose lives are within the part to set the terms of their union with the larger nation – which is in perennial question.

In a 1997 address to the Association for Canadian Studies Leslie Armour touched on the limits of rational pluralism, which he identified as the Canadian way of thinking – that is, its chief goal and preoccupation, owing to the fragmentation of Canadian society through its entire history. This isn't quite right. Canadian history seems to show rather that this way of thinking has emerged in the course of a long struggle between pluralists and those who want to make of us an undifferentiated whole, and have tried to enforce exclusion and assimilation. Ultimately this project cannot succeed, because it results only in resistance and war, or in vacuity. Armour goes on to say that "there does have to be a unity that is to be expressed. So there are cultural practices that seem strange to us but should surely be tolerated, and there are others that are not to be condoned" (22).

Armour adds, "the distinction has often been hard to make." The distinction, again, between those options that "can maintain plurality while truly expressing unity" and those that cannot. The premise here is equality of estimation as between all persons. It would be easy to bring forward a number of examples of traditional practices and views in which it is not easy to distinguish questions of difference (say, gender) from those of equality. It is well to be clear that what is compressed within the phase *rational pluralism* is in fact a program of ongoing world revolution in which every difference that can actually be reconciled to equality without being erased will be so reconciled – and those that cannot will indeed be erased.[223]

According to R. A. J. Phillips, who should have known, there was a conscious decision to avoid making of the Arctic a "special area" (read, reservation) in which government writ would run differently than elsewhere in the country. Rather, the newly attentive federal administration would replicate, over time, and without expensively duplicating personnel, the federal/provincial/municipal categories without necessarily planning for any of the territory to attain provincial status on the model of the prairie provinces (165).[224] Greater Canada would be just that: Canadian through and through in its institutions – except that this included, as Gordon Robertson noted in hindsight, the ultimate Canadian compromise, the minority stronghold, that is to say, a special area after all. Thus Nunavut, as Robertson saw it, was parted from the territories analogously to the separation of the Canadas under the British North America Act, which provided French

America with an administrative unit for the defense of its language and culture (208).

The proclamation of Nunavut offered to southern-dwelling Canadians a response to Aboriginal political insistence more in keeping with their rather inflated conception of their own moral excellence than previous, often highly aggressive projects. And there we rest, although the large expenditures and disappointments of Nunavut (of which most in southern Canada know little apart from the regular horror stories about dope and suicide in the news media) and the dislocations of climate change will surely lead to another round of recriminations.[225]

In 2007 Mary Cousins, born Panigusiq in Pond Inlet, voyager on the *St. Roch*, student in Hamilton, interpreter on the *Howe*, participant in the first meeting of Inuit Tapirisat of Canada, first editor of *Inuktitut*, goodwill ambassador to Ghana, artist, teacher, et cetera, died in Ottawa. Her family used the letters page of the *Nunatsiaq News* on May 11, 2007, to thank all those who had supported their mother during her final illness and offered their condolences on her death.

The editors printed nine other letters in that issue. They offer a cross-section of the situation. One was in memory of another elder, Jackoosie Iqalluq, a High Arctic relocatee, or exile as the Inuit lobby styles them, who re-relocated to Kuujjuaq in 1977, and who died a week before Cousins. The remaining eight letters testified to the transfer of authority, if not to the great success of its holders. (Five were signed "Name withheld by request.") One had to do with the registration of former residential school students in a Nunavut government-sponsored survey. One was about a controversy over the regulatory system as it affected mining investment choices in the territory. One was from the recently fired executive director of the Nunavut Water Board, who had a few things to get off his chest with regard to the efficiency or lack of it in the Nunavut public service. One was from a pair of concerned bureaucrats who feared that the premier, the government of Nunavut and the regional Kitikmeot Inuit Association were preparing to sacrifice environmental protections to mining interests. One was from an Inuk who thought that, contrary to the views of many elders and hunters, the polar bear quotas should be reduced. One was from the head of the Nunavik Police Association, who wanted to correct some inaccuracies in an article about negotiations with the employer. One was about the absence of Inuktitut from the Iqaluit Post Office, where there was not a single sign in the official language, nor a single speaker of it to serve the public. And one was about alcohol and its effects on families whose children are abused due to drink and who themselves turn to alcohol or other substances to obtain the same effects.

Nunavut counts about thirty thousand people in twenty-six villages. Nunavik has about twelve thousand in another fourteen. These entities differ in their political arrangements: one is a self-governing territory; the other has been promised regional government within the province of Quebec, seated at Kuujjuaq. Many members of both are strong swimmers on the internet and quite cosmopolitan in outlook, meeting and collaborating with colleagues and friends in all the circumpolar lands. Nunavut is the apogee of the welfare state, presumably the *ultima Thule* of its expansion, in terms of the kinds of services offered and the degree of subsidy required to do so. Some liken the economy to that of a rentier state, like those of the Arabian Gulf that receive most of their funds from the sale of oil alone. About ninety percent of the Nunavut government's funds are transfers from the federal government. It would seem that with the northern regions, as with others in the country having a great deal of sublime geography and not much in the way of revenue-generating economic activity, the Canadian state is prepared to pay very well to keep its sovereignty intact and continuous from the Alaskan boundary to Cape Spear, and to go on paying indefinitely. Whether the Nunavummiut can or will remain in dependency for as long is another matter. It seems more likely that young people will begin to depart, as they did from Newfoundland for many years before offshore oil pumping got properly underway.

Apart from patriotic satisfaction and lordly pride in the majesty of our leaseholdings and the vastness of our rental portfolio, the return, if ever there is one, on this expenditure is evidently judged worth the wait, but there does not appear to be any discursive account as to what that return is expected to be. Nor is anyone making odious comparisons between the funds disbursed to keep Nunavummiut in heating oil and Pepsi with alternative uses for the money. (No doubt there is an inventory of the known mineral resources and their potential for profit.) There is a grandeur about Canada (a grandeur with a much lighter admixture of fear since the advent of the helicopter and radio-assisted search-and-rescue crews) that is owing not only to the scale of it but also to the extravagant, not to say mad, pretensions of the Canadian state, through which we have undertaken to provide similar levels of public services in all parts of Our and Their Land. However, even as large and sparsely populated a region as Newfoundland has five hundred thousand inhabitants, extensive roadways, and affordable plane and ferry connections to the rest of the world, and is therefore accessible to most. The towns of Nunavut and Nunavik are not easily reached, and will remain Their Land in a way that Newfoundland and Quebec, let alone the other provinces and territories, do not.

EPILOGUE

Between 1952 and 1963, thirty-seven Inuit patients died in Hamilton and were buried there in Woodland Cemetery, at first in graves unmarked except in cemetery records.

Sometime between 1963 and the end of 1989, when Charlie Crow came from Sanikiluaq with his wife and daughters to visit, a wooden stake was set to mark each place. Crow, at that time the member of the legislative assembly for his district, had been in Hamilton before – not for tuberculosis treatment (although he had had that experience also), but as a boarder at the San while waiting to attend the Ontario School for the Blind in Brantford. Six of those buried at Woodland were from the Belcher Islands. With the assistance of Brian Burrows, who had been Anglican chaplain at the San, and who read the Anglican committal, Crow performed a simple ceremony for each of the six. Also attending was a city alderman, John Smith, who told the local newspaper that he was attempting to raise money toward the cemetery manager's project of erecting a monument on the site (James).

Nothing followed until 1994, when Connie Merkosak, a young woman from Pond Inlet, came to town to spend the summer with Pauline Hewak and Jerry Apanasowicz, teachers whom she had come to know during their time in the North. While in Hamilton, Merkosak visited the grave of her grandfather, Joanassie Kippuge. Aware of the stalled proposal for a memorial stone at the site, Merkosak's hosts contacted Paul Wilson, a columnist for the *Hamilton Spectator*, who took up the story. Wilson reported that a design had been commissioned but the money to carry through was absent. This publicity had the desired effect, for the City of Hamilton quickly approved a contribution of $16,500, about a third of the cost, with the remainder coming from Ottawa, Yellowknife and other donors.

The following year a granite stela, the work of Nicholas Neu, was erected close to the graves. The monument was ornamented with relief carvings suggested by soapstone work on display at the San, surmounted by an owl, and bore the names of the dead in both syllabic and Roman script.[226]

A dedication ceremony took place on June 11, 1995 (Ralph Holland Wilson, 181). The Anglican Church was there, as were the RCMP, along with thirty Inuit – among them Ann Hanson, at that time between her appointments as deputy commissioner of the Northwest Territories and commissioner of Nunavut. Also attending were nurses who had worked with Inuit patients at the San.[227]

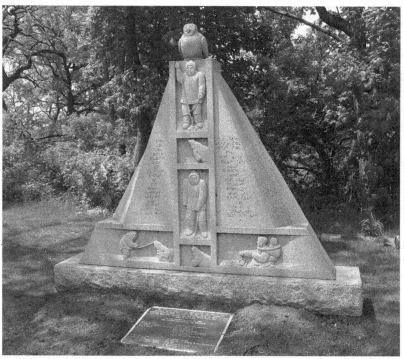

Monument to the Inuit buried in Woodland Cemetery, Hamilton.
© Bob Mesher, private collection.

In March 2005 Muktar Akumalik and his younger brother Percy came south to visit the grave of their father. With them were Joanasie

Akumalik, Muktar's adopted son, and Joanasie's son-in-law, Richard. Percy had been to the grave before, in 1984. Muktar had been intending for a long time to make the trip, and Percy was anxious for him to do so, but the flight and other travel expenses were very dear.

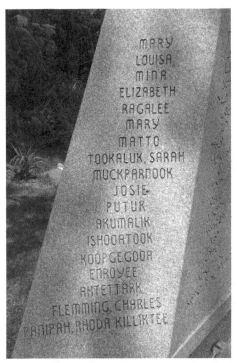

The names of those buried in Hamilton are inscribed on the monument. Shown here is the partial list, which appears on the south face of the monument. A similar inscription appears on the north face.
© Bob Mesher, private collection.

Because an acquaintance of mine planned to make a film for television about the evacuations, he had been speaking with David Poisey, an Inuk at Pangnirtung, who might direct the documentary. Poisey alerted us to the impending arrival of Muktar and his brother, and we were able to meet and talk with them while they were in Hamilton.

My acquaintance and I met with the four men at the film producer's house on the eve of their visit to the cemetery and again the following morning, in a room at the Indigenous Studies department at nearby McMaster University.

Muktar's father, Akumalik, had died in Hamilton after coming out of Arctic Bay in 1956, and is buried in Woodland cemetery, near the Inuit monument. (Simpson, reporting on the 1953 medical patrol's stop in Arctic Bay, said that fifty-four were x-rayed there, and that "there was no serious illness and E5-606 Akoomalik who was the only seriously ill patient in 1952 had greatly improved."[228]) The cemetery keepers know the location of each Inuit grave, and are able to guide visitors to the very plot where their relative lies.

Speaking through Joanasie, the brothers said that their father had been a leader in the community. He arranged matters so that one son would hunt food for the dogs, the other caribou for clothing. Since he had a boat, the family would also hunt seal through the summer and cache the meat for the dogs. In winter, they would instigate meetings of the people at his camp to talk through and resolve any problems in the community. This harmony would ensure that hunting continued to go well. He was very generous and providential. If there was sickness with any persons, he would immediately go to them and inquire as to what they might need. No one was ever left to go hungry.

When Akumalik became ill, he recalled that one day long before he had been outside the camp by himself when three large people approached him. One of them kicked him in the stomach. Because this was an act of shamanism, he forgot about it until much later when he fell sick. Three times he went out to Winnipeg for treatment. On one occasion, he went to Arctic Bay to meet the *Nascopie*, on what turned out to be that ship's last trip. On the third occasion he somehow came to be sent to Mountain Sanatorium, and there he died. But for many months the family had expected him to return. Percy learned of his death on taking a patient in to Hall Beach, where there was a nursing station. At that time he and Muktar were not together. Percy was eighteen when their father left, Muktar twenty-eight. There were three brothers and three sisters. Their mother also was away for three years, to hospital in Brandon, so for a time neither parent was present. When Akumalik was gone, the brothers no longer acted in a brotherly manner. Percy was living with his sister, his mind was a blank with regard to their father and he felt he had no other siblings.

Because Akumalik wished his children to become independent, he discouraged them from coming to him with complaints about others. When his father was gone, Percy felt alone, and had no home and went unfed. This troubled him for many years. He grew up angry and did not know any better: anger was the only way of life he knew. He had to break down to nothing before that could change. Eventually an elder from Pond Inlet told him where his father was buried. In 1984 he went south to place flowers at his father's grave and with them a note in which he wrote, *Father, they denied me food, I had no home.* Since coming down he had wanted Muktar to make the trip also, which finally he was able to do.

When Akumalik was ill, Muktar went in to where he was resting, and his father told him to take a pair of sealskin pants when he went out. But Muktar was so focused on his anxiety over his father's illness that he forgot to take the pants. At the grave, he was able to tell his father that he had forgotten. The brothers were able to look back to the time of their childhood, before the family fell apart and when they still acted as brothers. They embraced and wept.

In conclusion, Muktar said that now he would be better able to assist others with his counsel as an elder. "If two people have a problem," he said, "I cannot help them if I myself have problems. Perhaps I will even make problems between them. In general, many of the older people have problems that make it difficult for them to give guidance to the young as they should. There are unsettled matters in many people's hearts. When I go back I will talk about the experience of coming here. Some will like it and some will not. There is also to be a family reunion in the fall, and I will talk about this there."

As to the father's soul, the brothers felt that because he lived his religion and helped others, he had gone to heaven. If they act in their lives as he did, they will meet him there.

ACKNOWLEDGEMENTS

Researching a book of this sort is an experience of prolonged uncertainty and confusion, punctuated by the odd moment of clarification soon occluded by new confusions, leading one to an ever-greater appreciation for one's own ignorance and incapacity. And then you stop. Fortunately, I found plenty of help along the way, or I wouldn't be writing these words.

I am grateful to the many individuals who gave their time to recall for a stranger the details of a distant chapter of their lives: Fred Lee, Jr., Murray Ault, the late Kathe Neuman and Eka Berends, Bob Mesher, Hilda Ferrier, Nancy Anilniliak, Ann Van der Heiden, Gerda Selway and others. Thanks also to Ebba Olofsson and Bob Mesher, who shared thoughts when our research paths intersected.

I owe a special debt to the late Johanna Rabinowitz (née van der Woerd), who spent many hours telling me of her experiences on the *C.D. Howe*, and of her life before and after. Her donation greatly enlarged the photographic record of the Eastern Arctic Patrol in the Archives of the Hamilton Health Sciences and the Faculty of Health Sciences at McMaster University.

For easing some perplexities and adding others I wish to thank Peter Midgley and the anonymous readers for the University of Alberta Press, who undertook the onerous task of reading early, very thick, drafts. Although that relationship did not last, their work was very helpful to me.

The staff at Library and Archives Canada, the departmental library at Health Canada and the Local History & Archives of the Hamilton Public Library were grand, as were Anne McKeage at the Archives of the Hamilton Health Sciences and the Faculty of Health Sciences, and John Tagg at the Godfrey L. Gale Archives and Museum, West Park Healthcare Centre in Toronto.

The editors of this work, Jen Hale and Ashley Hisson, had a lot to do. I thank them. If faults remain it's because either I don't know any better, or because I refused to heed their good advice.

Finally, I wish to dedicate this book to my mother, who was there when the episode described here was unfolding, and who persisted in bringing this matter to the attention of an indifferent and skeptical son; and to the memory of the thirty-seven northern sojourners in the south who never returned home from Hamilton. Much has been changed since those days; much remains to do.

NOTES

PREFACE

1   Historicists both assume and deny human bodily and logical continuity (by logic here I mean arithmetic, duality and the complementarity that underlies dualities and makes them both stable and unstable) against which they assert the claim of "reason's inevitable parochiality" (Carl Page). According to philosopher Jerry Fodor:

> The idea that cognition saturates perception belongs with…the idea in the philosophy of science that one's observations are comprehensively determined by one's theories; with the idea in anthropology that one's values are comprehensively determined by one's culture; with the idea in sociology that one's epistemic commitments, including especially one's science, are comprehensively determined by one's class affiliations; and with the idea in linguistics that one's metaphysics is comprehensively determined by one's syntax. All these ideas imply a sort of relativistic holism: because perception is saturated by cognition, observations by theory, values by culture, science by class and metaphysics by language, rational criticism of scientific theories, ethical value, metaphysical world-views, or whatever can take place only within the framework of assumptions – as a matter of geographical, historical, or sociological accident, the interlocutors happen to share. What you can't do is criticize the framework…I think that relativism is very probably false. What it overlooks, to put it briefly and crudely, is the fixed structure of human nature." (Quoted in Cain, 204)

INTRODUCTION

2   *Hamilton Spectator*, April 19, 1950, in Mountain Sanatorium Scrapbook, vol. 2, 1950–1961, 7, Local History & Archives, Hamilton Public Library (hereafter cited as LH&A).

3   "Delayed by Hurricane 51 Cree Patients Arrive," *Hamilton Spectator*, October 27, 1954, in Mountain Sanatorium Scrapbook, vol. 2, 1950–1961, 67, LH&A.

4   *Hamilton Health Association Bulletin* (March 1961), Archives of the Hamilton Health Sciences and the Faculty of Health Sciences, McMaster University, Hamilton Health Sciences Fonds, Hamilton Health Association Subfonds (hereafter cited as Archives of HHS & FHS).

5   Anne McKeage, "Research of Inuits," is a fact sheet for researchers prepared by the archivist of the Archives of HHS & FHS on January 16, 1990, which contains a summary of the patient count year by year drawn from the Hamilton Health Association annual reports.

6   But old attitudes lingered. Ian Mosby has published an account of medical studies conducted among residential school students between 1942 and 1952 by health workers who should have been helping, not just observing. The researchers, finding that the children in a number of these places were malnourished, provided extra nutrition to some while withholding this benefit from others in order to observe the effects. See Ian Mosby, "Administering Colonial Science: Nutrition Research and Human Biomedical Experimentation in Aboriginal Communities and Residential Schools, 1942–1952," *Histoire sociale/Social history* 46, no. 91 (Mai-May 2013): 145–72.

7   See Eggleston, 352, for a summary of what occurred during "reconstruction":

> During 1952, some 1,900 machine tools valued at about 12.3 million were delivered to Canadian defence construction plants, and new orders in the same period were placed for 1203 new machines, valued at 6.3 million . . . Between August 1945 and the end of 1951 over 1500 entirely new manufacturing establishments have begun operating in Canada. These represented an investment of about $6000 million; they provided employment for about 75,000 people; and in 1951 their production was worth 700 million . . . In 1950, Canada spent over 1.4 billion on new machinery and equipment, and in 1951, upwards of 1.8 billion. This runs at the rate of eight or nine percent of the total national expenditure on all goods and services. Only once before, 1926–1930, has investment in this field even approached such a proportion of the national income.

8   See also Bruce Muirhead, *The Development of Postwar Canadian Trade Policy: The Failure of the Anglo-European Option* (Montreal: McGill-Queen's University Press, 1992). Muirhead goes carefully through the particulars. Canadian readers will emerge from this account feeling a bitter pride that our negotiators got us through yet another fine milling between Mom and Uncle.

9   The Americans had already, on three occasions crucial to Canadian financial health, acted upon a perceived community of interests, or, to put it more bluntly, had pulled us out of the shit when we had gotten stuck there owing to our fond eagerness to keep faith with the British – who certainly did not reciprocate the loyalty of the lesser breeds. The first bit of bother occurred during the First World War. Shortly after Vimy, in the spring of 1917, the British told Ottawa that it could no longer pay for what it was getting from Canada. If the orders were

to be maintained, then the Canadian government would have to finance them. Unfortunately this was a two-sided problem. Since Canada was importing much in the way of tools and munitions components from the States in order to make war goods for Britain, the more Canadians gave to the Brits, the deeper into debt we would go with the Americans. Canada therefore needed to borrow from the US to buy in the US to supply Britain – but there was a ban of foreign private borrowing in the States. Ottawa convinced the Americans to make an exception for Canada and some months later extended a loan of US dollars to the British, which they used to pay for Canadian material and which Canadians in turn re-spent in the US (Granatstein, 14).

Twenty-five years later, the same thing happened again. Supplying Britain, at war with Germany, was again creating a Canadian deficit with the still neutral Americans. Franklin Roosevelt devised Lend-Lease as a means of coming to the aid of the British. Unfortunately, Lend-Lease gave its beneficiary every incentive to switch orders from Canada to the US. Again, the answer was to have the Americans charge exports going to Canada for purposes of manufacturing war material for Britain to the British Lend-Lease account. Better still, if the US would buy raw material in Canada to balance Canadian purchases in the States, everything would be rosy all around – and the Americans kindly obliged. Finally, in the spring of 1948, this same sad scenario came around once again. Once more Canada was financing British imports from the US with a loan, while running a steep deficit with the US. Once more the Americans, this time under the Marshall Plan (the Economic Cooperation Act) provided dollars to Britain, which could be used in turn to buy in Canada.

10   A stark example of the economic reconciliation of war and peace is offered by Frigidaire, a subsidiary of General Motors with plants in Canada. In 1952 the company built a ten-acre plant on Scarborough's Golden Mile, whence flowed a thousand appliances a day (mostly refrigerators and stoves). The technically demanding compressors for the fridges however continued to be made at the old plant in the Leaside neighbourhood of Toronto, whose workers now also turned out turbine blades for the engines of jet fighters (see Eggleston, 352).

11   This change was prepared in the fifties and carried though in the sixties. See José Eduardo Igartua, *The Other Quiet Revolution: National Identities in English Canada, 1945–71* (Vancouver: University of British Columbia Press, 2006).

12   Many of the contradictions and confusions are seen in high relief in Ottawa's much-studied northward relocation "experiments" of 1953 and after. The experiments were in rehabilitation. The Inuit as a people were thought by Euro-Canadian observers to have become overly reliant on outside help to get by. This help was expensive for Ottawa and demoralizing for the Inuit themselves. It would be better for both if the Inuit would continue the old ways of gaining a living – in new territories if necessary. The choice of a particular territory to be colonized was probably strongly influenced by the uncertain status of Canadian claims to sovereignty in the High Arctic, although this is officially denied. Shelagh D. Grant went through the archives very thoroughly to rebut an earlier research effort by a

government-employed consultant that denied the importance of anxieties about sovereignty in the minds of the relocators. She said also that "by March 1954, the reference to 'the experiment' virtually disappeared from written documents, abruptly and without explanation. While there is no evidence of willful wrong-doing or malicious intent, the nature of the arrangements indicated apparent ignorance of the responsibilities as set out in the United Nations Declaration of Human Rights (1948)" (Grant, 13). "Experiment" certainly was in fashion, how-ever. R. A. J. Phillips said in 1955, before he became chief of the Arctic Division of Northern Affairs, "To think of 9,000 Eskimos as a laboratory experiment and to give the imagination full rein on what might be done to improve the culture is easy when travelling in the company of so effective and so enthusiastic an organizer of public health as Dr. Willis [General Superintendent of Northern Health]. He bubbles with ideas on every phase of Eskimo life from housing to hygiene." See R. A. J. Phillips, Eastern Arctic Patrol 1955 Montreal to Resolute, September 1955. Library and Archives Canada, Record Group 22, vol. 319, file 40-2-20, pt. 4, 106.

13   A good discussion of "Social Welfare and Social Crisis in the Eastern Arctic" appears in Tester and Kulchyski, 43–101.

14   "Eskimo Polar Bear Hunter Agile with Artificial Legs," *Edmonton Journal*, repro-duced by *Camsell Arrow* in January 1968. See Charles Camsell History Committee, 156.

15   "Aftermath," *The Beaver*, December 1953, 34.

16   Library and Archives Canada (LAC), Record Group (RG) 29, vol. 2874, file 851-1-12, pt. 1A.

17   LAC, RG 29, vol. 2874, file 851-1-12, pt. 1B.

ONE: THE RATIONALE

18   Archives of HHS & FHS, RG Board, 1952.

19   Archives of HHS & FHS, RG Board, 1953.

20   Archives of HHS & FHS, RG Board, 1954.

21   Moore to Young, 24 March 1953. LAC, RG 22, vol. 254, file 40-8-1, pt. 3.

22   The reasons for this divergence are discussed in Georgina D. Feldberg, *Disease and Class: Tuberculosis and the Shaping of Modern North American Society* (New Brunswick, NJ: Rutgers University Press, 1995).

23   This may be the origin of the view expressed by some Inuit that they were experi-mented upon in the hospitals.

24 The remark was made by Allen Roses, Vice-President of Genetics, who on the same occasion told *The Independent* that drugs for cancer work in only a quarter of the recipients; drugs for migraines, osteoporosis and arthritis in about half. What this may mean is simply that there a great many substances that have been approved for sale as having more possible benefits than harms. In the case of anti-TB medications circa 1950, the potential benefits of the drug were so great that withholding it because the full range of individual response was unknown would have been very difficult to justify; providing the drug in a closely monitored setting was much easier.

25 Extract from *Annual Report of the Mountain Sanatorium 1953* reproduced in *Mountain Views*, the mimeographed patient newsletter, Archives of HHS & FHS.

26 Grygier writes, "Perhaps the main reason [for the harms they inflicted] was one of which many of the government workers may not even have been aware, because they were so much a part of it, so immersed in it, that it seemed entirely normal; namely, the prevailing colonial, paternalistic attitudes of the period in which they had been reared" (177). This view, that colonialism was in them because they were saturated with it, is ultimately more forgiving of the wrongs of the past and more convenient for the living beneficiaries of those wrongs than is the moralistic stance that I prefer as truer to the perpetual human experience of finding oneself obliged to choose not between good and evil, but between combinations of both.

27 Researchers requesting government documents held at Library and Archives Canada are advised of the requirement to supress names or identifying information (such as disc numbers) in citing any of the material, and any requested copies are "anonymized" by staff before they are released. Similarly, of course, with hospital archives.

28 Training and deployment of these individuals is described in detail in John Adair, Kurt W. Deuschle and Clifford R. Barnett, *The People's Health: Medicine and Anthropology in a Navajo Community* (New York: Appleton-Century-Crofts, 1970). Unfortunately this innovation occurred within the terms of a contract between Cornell University Medical College and the federal bureaucracy. At the end of the contract, the Department of Health, Education and Welfare re-entered the field and took on the health visitors, but under existing civil-service job descriptions, which effectively nullified their training. Adair, Deuschle and Barnett comment: "Programs that are welcomed in less developed countries are often defeated due to conflicts within the society of the donor . . . The designing of services which properly fit the needs of a society as different from ours as that of the Navajo requires a modification in our institutions and in the customary procedures of our own professionals. That is the most difficult part of the job. Innovation requires changes in both the donor and the recipient societies" (144).

29 The Euro-American physicians were able to work their way into a complementary position with Navajo hand tremblers (diagnosticians) and singers (therapists) since their techniques were not really full substitutes for each other. Once this was

recognized by both parties, the work was shared out, according as the one or the other could demonstrate greater efficacy with any particular complaint.

30 Department of Health and Welfare Library, Medical Sciences Annual Review, Directorate Report INHS 1959.

31 Ibid.

TWO: POWERS

32 "Annual Trek to the North," *Shipping Register and Shipbuilding*, reproduced in "Clipped Comment," *North/Nord* 7, no. 4–5 (July–October 1960): 61.

33 For the ownership record, see the "Great Lakes Vessels Online Index," Bowling Green State University, accessed April 15, 2015, http://greatlakes.bgsu.edu/vessel/view/002654. For the use in Greenland, see Charles Maginley and Bernard Collin, *The Ships of Canada's Marine Services* (St. Catharines: Vanwell Publishing, 2001), 146.

34 John Willis, Preliminary Report of the Medical Party, "C.D. Howe," July 1955. LAC, RG 85, vol. 1903, file 1009-13, pt. 1.

35 Clearly this analysis must be continually renewed. A quick web search in May 2007 on the term *mass miniature radiography* yielded reports from Pakistan and Japan, widely different in their conclusions. Pakistan in 1997 was still sending a van around Karachi to screen school children, factory workers and the Afghani inhabitants of refugee camps. In Japan, as of 2002, fifty-four million people over the age of twenty-five were being x-rayed every year, but the number of cases found was quite small. Consequently the cost per case to find the disease was roughly five or six times greater than the cost to treat that case with two months hospitalization followed by four months of outpatient service.

36 George S. MacCarthy and Campbell Laidlaw, Report on the Southern Half of the Eastern Arctic Patrol, September 28, 1945. LAC, RG 29, vol. 2874, file 851-1-12, part 1A, 4.

37 Harry W. Lewis, Final Report of X-Ray Survey of Eskimos Eastern Arctic 1946, n.d. LAC, RG 29, vol. 2874, file 851-1-12, pt. 1-B.

38 Ibid.

39 Labrecque to Leroux, 22 December 1951. LAC, RG 29, vol. 2875, file 851-1-12, pt. 3A.

40 Lee to Moore, 25 January 1958. LAC, RG 29, vol. 2875, file 851-1-12, pt. 6.

41   Surprisingly, he also suggested a "photo timing unit, with appropriate cassette, to help produce films of uniform density." The photometer, a device to automatically halt radiation when correct exposure of the film was complete, had been standard equipment since about 1949. Exposure time and development time are directly related. On the *Howe*, the need to reduce exposure cannot be made by extending development time, because so many persons had to be screened in so short a period.

42   *Annual Report Eastern Arctic Patrol 1958*, n.d. LAC, RG 29, vol. 2875, file 852-2-12, pt. 6.

43   Lee to Moore, 25 January 1958. LAC, RG 29, vol. 2875, file 851-1-12, pt. 6.

44   *Medical Services Annual Review 1959*, Indian and Northern Health Services, Medical Services Directorate Health and Welfare Canada. However, J. E. Labrecque had already written in a letter from 1951 that "we took the liberty of checking the patients actually hospitalized, against last year's report of the survey and we may say that the X-ray diagnosis was accurate in 100% of the 36 cases in hospital who had had a film taken on that occasion." Labrecque to Leroux, 22 December 1951. LAC, RG 29, vol. 2875, file 851-1-12, pt. 3A.

45   Moore to Cunningham, Medical Services for and Hospitalization of Eskimos, 16 June 1953. LAC, RG 85, vol. 1072, file 252-3.

46   Bent G. Sivertz, Eastern Arctic Patrol First Part of Voyage, August 27, 1954. Secret and Confidential Documents. LAC RG 85, vol. 1903, file 1009-13, pt. 1.

47   Arctic Medical Survey Parties, Summer 1955. Health Canada Departmental Library, Department of National Health and Welfare, Indian and Eskimo Health Services, RC958.c2 E13 1955.

48   Ibid.

49   Admitted to southern hospitals: 524; discharged to home: 599; born in southern hospitals: 26; died: 10. (*Medical Services Annual Review 1959*, 70. Health Canada Departmental Library, Department of National Health and Welfare, Medical Services Directorate, Indian and Northern Health Services, RA 184/C212.)

50   Willis, Preliminary Report.

51   H. B. Sabean, Extracts from Report by Dr. H. B. Sabean on the Medical Work of the Eastern Arctic Patrol, 1957. LAC, RG 85, vol. 452, file 201-1, pt. 37; Grygier, 99.

52   R. A. J. Phillips, Report of a Trip to the Central Arctic, April 21, 1955. Secret and Confidential Documents. LAC, RG 85, vol. 1903. file 1009-13, pt. 1.

53   Ibid.

54   Ibid.

55   R. A. J. Phillips, Eastern Arctic Patrol 1955 Montreal to Resolute, September 1955. LAC, RG 22, vol. 319, file 40-2-20, pt. 4, 42.

56   On retiring as deputy director general of Information Canada in 1972, he spent five years as founding executive director of Heritage Canada, an organization he and his wife had set up with others to play a role like that of the British and American trusts for the preservation of the national patrimony. See Brian Anthony, "A Tribute to R.A.J. Phillips," *Heritage: The Magazine of the Heritage Canada Foundation* (Fall 2003). According to a daughter, Phillips wrote daily but largely eschewed the personal until his final years, when he began to write down some of the anecdotes that made his reputation as a raconteur. This material was recorded on an unreliable computer onto antiquated diskettes and at present remains in that form only.

57   Marcus was able to establish – by working through memoranda and correspondence, and by personal conversation – that the bureaucrats used Mowat essentially to deflect the blame for their own poor decisions onto the RCMP, who had refused to assist Mowat in his research. But more importantly, the administrators felt that publicity on the scale that Mowat was able to stimulate would improve their chances of increased funding and so their ability to carry out more of their plans quickly. Mowat shared their wish for greater intervention and this was the basis of their co-operation. It should be noted, however, that the Northern Affairs people acknowledged that Mowat's information about conditions, gained on the ground, was better than theirs; and that their direct assistance during the writing of *The Desperate People* was confined to providing statistics and general information in response to Mowat's queries.

58   Willis, Preliminary Report.

59   Otto Schaefer, Preliminary Evaluation of the Eastern Arctic Survey 1964, n.d., in regard to the Planned Arctic Research Program 1964. LAC, RG 29, vol. 2876, file 851-1-12, pt. 7.

60   Ibid.

61   Phillips, Eastern Arctic Patrol 1955, 59.

62   Murray Ault, July 7, 1959, "Journal of a voyage on the *C. D. Howe* June 25– September 25, 1959," Personal Journal, in its author's possession.

63   Ibid.

64   R. Hayward, Report of the Eastern Arctic Patrol 1958 Resolute to Quebec City, 1958. LAC, RG 29, vol. 2875, file 851-1-12, pt. 6.

65 Others were Margery Hinds, the teacher and social worker variously at Fort McPherson, the Mackenzie River Delta, Port Harrison, Cape Dorset, the Sugluk Inlet and the Arctic Bay; Douglas Wilkinson the cinematographer; Charles Gimpel the art dealer; and Doctors Schaefer and Sabean.

66 When Spalding quit the company it was to take a degree at the University of Manitoba, and then another from McMaster with a thesis on Wordsworth, before returning to Northern service as a translator, lexicographer and fervent apostle of orthographic reform.

67 Hayward, Report of the Eastern Arctic Patrol 1958.

68 Johanna van der Woerd to parents, 1958, Rabinowitz Collection, Archives of HHS & FHS.

69 Willis, Preliminary Report, 11.

70 Ibid.

71 Marsh to Robertson, 4 February 1954. LAC, RG 22, vol. 254, file 40-8-1, pt. 4.

72 Willis, Preliminary Report, 11.

73 J. S. Willis to Director of Indian Health Services, Arctic Medical Survey Parties Summer, 195, April 20, 1955. Health Canada Departmental Library, Department of National Health and Welfare, Medical Services Directorate, Indian and Northern Health Services, RC958.c2 E13 1955.

74 In *High Arctic Venture*, Margery Hinds asserted that "for some years it has been the practice for two photographs to be taken of each individual's chest. One of these is processed and read on board, the other is taken out for processing" (177).

75 Willis, Preliminary Report.

76 Dr. Peter J. Moloney also came up with a reaction test to screen for people likely to react very strongly to the toxoid. These received a diluted version. Between 1925 and 1930 a team led by Dr. John G. FitzGerald conducted controlled studies in Hamilton, Brantford, Windsor and Toronto. After 1932 there were no new cases in Hamilton (Christopher J. Rutty, "Connaught and the Defeat of Diphtheria," *CONNTACT 9*, no. 1 [February 1996]: 11).

77 John Willis, "Northern Health: Problems and Progress," *North/Nord* 6, no. 5 (November/December 1959): 21–25.

78 BCG was a problem, because widespread use would destroy the tuberculin test. This was not a relevant consideration in so heavily tuberculized a population as the Inuit. However, the effects of BCG on a child under three would wear off by school age and the tuberculin test could be restored. BCG itself could be a test, but it took twenty-four hours to develop. The vaccine required cold chain

(temperature-controlled transport and storage) and was not simple to administer: drops had to be placed in scratches, lightly rubbed in, and then the scratch bandaged.

79   John Willis, Administrative Guide, Eastern Arctic Survey 1956, 108. Health Canada Departmental Library, Department of National Health and Welfare, INHS RC 958.C2 E13 1956.

80   Ibid. In 1959 there was an additional step at the end – cranial or facial measurements by an anthropologist, a Dr. Ochinski from Ottawa. Murray Ault, who sometimes assisted, thinks the purpose was to gauge the degree of mingling of Inuit and European heredity after some centuries of whaling activity in the north.

81   Ibid.

82   John Willis, Administrative Guide, Eastern Arctic Survey 1957, 2. Health Canada Departmental Library, Department of National Health and Welfare, INHS RC 958.C2 E13 1957.

83   Willis, Preliminary Report, 4.

84   Ibid., 6.

THREE: EVACUATION

85   R. N. Simpson, Eastern Arctic Patrol 1953, n.d. LAC, RG 85, vol. 316, file 201-1, pt. 29.

86   James Cantley, Memorandum for the Director, February 15, 1954. LAC, RG 85, vol. 316, file 201-1, pt. 29.

87   Willis, Preliminary Report, 8.

88   Willis, Second Preliminary Report, Eastern Arctic Patrol 1955. LAC, RG 29, vol. 2875, file 851-1-12, para. 21.

89   Ibid., para. 15.

90   H. B. Sabean, Extracts from Report.

91   Medical Services Annual Review 1959, 70. Department of Health and Welfare, Directorate Report 1959, INHS RA 184/C212 msb.

92   Willis, Preliminary Report, 4.

93 Phillips, Report on the Eastern Arctic Patrol 1955, 18–20. Library and Archives Canada/The Eastern Arctic Patrol/AMICUS 13499007/*Portion being used.*

94 Marsh to Robertson, 4 February 1954. LAC, RG 22, vol. 254, file 40-8-1, pt. 4. The date implies that the event took place the previous summer, that is, under Simpson, but Simpson's report on EAP 1953 does not mention any incidents at Lake Harbour (now Kimmirut) and does mention refusals of treatment elsewhere, which were accepted, so Marsh may be referring to another date, or reporting from a different perspective.

95 Phillips, Report on the Eastern Arctic Patrol 1955, 17.

96 Ibid., 63–65.

97 Ibid., 69.

98 Ibid., 71.

99 Ibid., 85.

100 Ibid., 73.

101 Ibid., 98.

102 Willis, Preliminary Report, 4.

103 Sivertz, Eastern Arctic Patrol First Part of Voyage.

104 LAC, RG 29, vol. 2875, file 851-1-12, pt. 6.

105 Ibid.

106 Sabean, Extracts from Report.

107 Leo Manning, Memorandum for Mr. Cantley, 2 March 1953. LAC, RG 85, vol. 1072, file 252-3, pt. 4.

108 J. Cantley to R. N. Simpson, 13 February 1953. LAC, RG 85, vol. 1072, file 252-3, pt. 4.

109 J. C. Osborne, 1950 Arctic Patrol Recommendations for Next Year, 1950. LAC, RG 29, vol. 2875, file 851-1-12, pt. 3A.

110 This is an informative article, marred by the authors' refusal to investigate the medical thinking or practice of the period. They know the question, that "it might well be asked to what extent hospitalization in the South was a necessity or reflected the culturally constructed norm for a profession which had, at the time, absolute control over every aspect of hospital treatment and administration" (137), but they

don't look into it. Since they know in advance that the doctor's decisions were culturally bound by colonialist, et cetera, there is nothing to investigate.

111 Manning, Memorandum for Mr. Cantley.

112 LAC, RG 22, vol. 254, file 40-8-1, pt. 3.

113 LAC, RG 85, vol. 316, file 201-1, pt. 29. This was repeated at least once more, as an article on the EAP produced by Phillips for *Canadian Geographical Journal* is illustrated with, among others, a photograph credited to him and captioned "Cape Dorset Eskimos listen to tape recordings made by neighbours who are in hospital in the south" (R.A.J. Phillips, "The Eastern Arctic Patrol," *Canadian Geographical Journal* 54 [May 1957]: 190–201).

114 LAC, RG 85, vol. 316, file 201-1, pt. 29.

115 Ibid.

116 Sivertz to Hinds, 26 November 1954. LAC, RG 22, vol. 319, file 40-2-20, pt. 4.

117 J. V. Jacobsen, Memorandum for the Director, June 21, 1955. LAC, RG 22, vol. 319, file 40-2-20, pt. 4.

118 In his report of that year's EAP, Sabean, the medical officer in charge, was appreciative of Banffy's work and stressed that her position was "indispensable" to the "actual mechanism of evacuation." He wrote, "Unfortunately, during the very early part of the trip full advantage of the welfare officer's assistance was not utilized; this was, I believe, partly because we had not yet sorted ourselves out enough to incorporate this new position into our thinking" (H. B. Sabean, Extracts from Report).

119 One wonders what became of these photographs.

120 R. C. Hastings, Report of Doctor R. C. Hastings, medical officer of the CGS *N.B. McLean* covering tour of the eastern arctic in 1945, n.d. LAC, RG 29, vol. 2874, file 851-1-12, pt. 1-B.

121 R. A. Gibson to P. E. Moore, December 7, 1945.

122 Ibid.

123 R. C. Hastings, Report.

124 Willis expressed this fear: "We have seen a number of Eskimos who are definitely in need of institutional care. The two children at Koartak [now Quaqtaq] are in such a state that they could be made into Newspaper dynamite. We must pray that our friend of the Vancouver Sun [presumably Stanley Burke, who had written critically of the *Howe*'s operations the year before] does not hear about them or cannot get to them with a camera." Willis, Preliminary Report, 16.

125 Phillips, Eastern Arctic Patrol 1955, 106.

126 Minutes of the Committee on Eskimo Affairs 1953. LAC, RG 22, vol. 254, file 40-8-1, pt. 3.

127 However, the testimony recorded by the Qikiqtani Truth Commission casts some doubt on this proposition, as a number of witnesses said that they had not previously talked about these matters in private or in public. In November 2006 an archivist at Library and Archives Canada familiar with Northern Affairs records said that two boxes of letters from the Inuit, in Inuktitut with English translation, were among the holdings, but these files were judged too sensitive for release. These may be some or all of the fifty-four letters examined by Tester, McNicoll and Irniq in preparing the article "Writing for Our Lives." However, those were written primarily from Hamilton and Brandon, MB, to Leo Manning and were not translated. In any case, Tester et al. supply no specific reference, complicating the task of following that particular trail.

128 *Medical Services Annual Review* 1959, Health and Welfare Canada Departmental Library, RA 184/ c212 msb.

129 LAC, RG 29, vol. 2875, file 851-1-12, pt. 6.

130 P. E. Moore to Regional Superintendent, Eastern Region, Medical Services, 5 March 1964. LAC, RG 29, vol. 2876, file 851-1-12, pt. 7.

131 Minutes of a Meeting to Discuss the Eastern Arctic Patrol 1966, December 15, 1965. LAC, RG 29, vol. 2876, file 851-1-12, pt. 7.

132 Norman Harper, X-ray survey – Eastern Arctic – Easter 1965, December 7, 1965.

133 Summary of Activities, Location: Eastern Arctic Patrol, July 12–September 24, 1965. LAC, RG 29, vol. 2876, file 851-1-12, pt. 7.

134 K. F. Butler to H. A. Procter, 12 March 1968. LAC, RG 29, vol. 2876, file 851-1-12, pt. 7.

FOUR: THE CAPTIVITY

135 "Canadian-Born Japanese Employed as Orderlies; Women Physicians Busy," *Hamilton Spectator*, August 3, 1943, in Mountain Sanatorium Scrapbook, vol. 1, LH&A.

136 H. Ewart, Biographical, Archives of HHS & FHS, box 102, accession 12.4.

137 Vallee to Valentine, 2 May 1958. LAC, RG 85, vol. 366, file 255-2-2.

138 Ibid.

139 According to Bernard Saladin d'Anglure, Frederiksen was something of a misfit, pugnacious and overly fond of contrasting his proficiency in Inuktitut with the limited skills of others. Also, his interests were out of the mainstream. Vallee and Valentine included Frederiksen in their anthology, with a piece about the soul.

140 Minister's Conference on Tuberculosis, Toronto, ON, March 15–16, 1962. The last Inuit patient was discharged from Mountain Sanatorium in 1963 and by the following year there were only forty TB patients in total at the San; in 1967, there were thirty-two.

141 "Extracts from the annual report of the Hamilton Health Association 1953," *Mountain Views*, n.d., Archives of HHS & FHS, Publications by Patients, box 92, accession 11.3.

142 Fumi Hirayama, "Strictly Business," *Mountain Views*, April 1951, Archives of HHS & FHS, Publications by Patients, box 92, accession 11.3.

143 "Canada's Status High Among Netherlanders," *Hamilton Spectator*, November 28, 1949, in Mountain Sanatorium Scrapbook, vol. 1, LH&A.

144 The record is probably held by James Tegeapak of Cambridge Bay, who arrived at the Camsell in 1952 and remained through 1963. See Charles Camsell History Committee, 106.

145 *To our Eskimo Patients* c. 1960–1965, Godfrey L. Gale Archives and Museum, West Park Healthcare Centre, Toronto (hereafter cited as Godfrey L. Gale Archives and Museum).

146 Ibid.

147 The reference to arsenic is not figurative; arsenic was an ingredient in Fowler's Solution, a tonic recommended in cases of TB of all sorts and even by William Osler, otherwise a noted "therapeutic nihilist" (Comroe). It was supposed to stimulate the body's resistance to the bacillus.

148 One would think that the percentage overall of patients undergoing the operation would be more relevant, but this may be an instance of last resort applied to hopeless cases, medical futility as we say, in which case the information would not be about the value of the procedure but the cultural constraints that shaped the doctor-patient relationship, hence decisions about intervention.

149 Reverse of an undated photograph, Archives of HHS & FHS, photographs, box 81, accession 10.1.

150 An article from December 1, 1956, in the *Globe and Mail* has Poag saying that no patient made more than $500 a year, but can this be accurate? What could one

patient have been doing that would bring in $500 when all the others combined made only $8,000?

151 Archives of HHS & FHS, Publications by Patients, box 92, accession 11.3.

152 "Delayed by Hurricane 51 Cree Patients Arrive," *Hamilton Spectator*, October 29, 1954, in Mountain Sanatorium Scrapbook, vol. 2, 1950–1961, LH&A.

153 *Hamilton Spectator*, December 11, 1954, in Mountain Sanatorium Scrapbook, vol. 2, 1950–1961, LH&A.

154 The Aboriginal syllabary, of which Inuktitut syllabics is a subset, was born out of controversy because it signified Euro-Canadian accommodation to Aboriginal culture. This was recognized and resisted at the moment of creation by James Evans at Rice Lake Ontario around 1831. Protestant missionaries identified Christianity with English, and preferred to convey the true religion in its native tongue. Second best was to offer the Word in Aboriginal languages in Romanic script, since this would help in the eventual acquisition of English. Evans's approach, begun during his time among the Ojibwa, assigned one character to each syllable, and so could be learnt in a few days. The innovation was not approved by his superiors, but after 1840, now transferred to Norway House, MB, he tried again, this time with Cree, and modelling his forms on Pitman shorthand and embossed scripts for the blind. In the fifties the script was carried to James Bay and adapted to Inuktitut, and after 1876, went with Edmund Peck to Ungava and Baffin Island. After many vicissitudes, Inuktitut syllabics is now available in a 16-bit Unicode font, and remains the preferred script in Nunavut and Nunavik.

155 *Mountain Views*, August 1955, Archives of HHS & FHS, Publications by Patients, box 92, accession 11.3.

156 Ibid.

157 Ibid.

158 Ibid.

159 Joanasie Salamonie to Marion MacKnight, n.d., postmark 1997, Archives of HHS & FHS, Sylvia James Papers, box 114.9, accession 2006.16.12.

160 At one point, the (rather delusory) preference for assimilation had gone so far that the resettlement of large numbers in the South was contemplated. It was expected that growth would make some fraction of the population surplus in the North. A pilot project involving ex-patients was mooted and Hamilton listed among the possible sites for this trial. The notion was that Inuit who had already become familiar with southern life were likely candidates for fuller cultural integration (see Tester and Kulchyski, 312). Although a few discharged patients did stay in the South, almost all returned home.

161 Minutes of the Mountain Sanatorium School Board meeting, January 7, 1955, Archives of HHS & FHS, RG Board.

162 Ibid., February 11, 1957.

163 Dr. H. Ewart, Medical Superintendent, Chedoke Hospital, 1947–1970, February 5, 1980, Archives of HHS & FHS, History of Medicine, Oral History Collection, box 26, McMaster Medical, file 2.

164 The occasion was a one-day "field trip" of medical researchers, archivists and museologists to the former San buildings, organized by Emily Farrell, a doctoral candidate in the Anthropology Department at McMaster University.

165 Minutes of the Mountain Sanatorium School Board meeting, February 14, 1955, Archives of HHS & FHS, RG Board.

166 Ibid., April 10, 1956.

167 Ibid., June 26, 1956.

168 Kingsley Brown, "New Eskimo Primer," *Hamilton Spectator*, September 12, 1956, Archives of HHS & FHS, Newsclips 1936–1957, box 72, accession 9.1.

169 Ibid.

170 Sarah Ekoomiak, an interpreter for the shipborne EAP in the early sixties, learned syllabics as a teenage TB patient at Moose Factory General Hospital. "When I was in the hospital I really wanted to write to my Dad. I was so close to my Dad. I asked the next bed lady, can you help teach me how to write Inuktitut? She would write two letters on a paper. She gave it to me. I tried to read it for her. Then she gave me two more letters, then three, four letters. She'd write to me and I'd answer back. Then I started to write letters to my Dad." This was the beauty of the system: easy to learn in a short time (Ekoomiak and Flynn-Burhoe).

171 Within ten years, Bernard Saladin d'Anglure had begun the program in Nunavik of having Nunavimmiut write letters to posterity, as it were, which resulted in the production of four thousand pages of first-hand ethnography.

172 Minutes of the Mountain Sanatorium School Board meeting, February 11, 1957, Archives of HHS & FHS, RG Board.

173 *Globe and Mail*, July 20, 1957. This title does not appear in Robin McGrath's bibliography of Inuit publications and ephemera. Since *Northern Lights and Shadows* may have been the embryo of *Inuktitut* magazine, whose first editor was Mary Panigusiq and so an early bloom in Inuit literary history, it would be very welcome if a few copies could be located.

174 Vallee to Valentine, 2 May 1958. LAC, RG 85, vol. 366, file 255-2-2.

175 J. David Ford, *Globe and Mail*, November 15, 1952. LAC, RG 22, vol. 254, file 40-8-1, pt. 3.

176 Helen Elliot Goglinsky, "The Lesson of David Mikeyook," *Globe and Mail*, December 20, 1952, Archives of HHS & FHS, Newsclips 1937–1957, box 72, accession 9.1.

177 I. Deroose, "The Strep Wagon," quoted in Larmour, 46.

178 H. Ewart, General, Anon, "The San Song," Archives of HHS & FHS, box 101, accession 12.3.

179 Alan H. Bailey, "Missouri San – Ozark," *Mountain Views*, November 1952, Archives of HHS & FHS, Publications by Patients, box 92, accession 11.3.

180 Harry Rubin, "Dat Dam Gastric," *Mountain Views*, June 1950, Archives of HHS & FHS, Publications by Patients, box 92, accession 11.3.

181 Unsigned and undated translation, Archives of HHS & FHS, Sylvia James, Inuit Patients, box 9, accession 202.13. On the first of these occasions, Sylvia James recalled, she made the mistake of playing these messages over the PA system, with the result that some of the children believed their parents were in the corridors and were very upset when they found it was not so.

182 "I'll always remember my first trip to Mount Hope airport on a hot humid day to see a group of patients flown in from near the Arctic circle. Their clothes were heavy and dirty and *smelly* and they were sick and exhausted. Then I saw in spite of all this an Eskimo herding his family together and joking and laughing with the interpreter. Imagine if you can their feelings on being bundled into ambulances, shot up in hospital elevators, given baths and pajamas and put to bed" (Sylvia James, manuscript notes for a talk, date illegible, Archives of HHS & FHS, Inuit Patients, box 9, accession 202.13).

183 "Our Cover Girl Maggie Hatuk," *50th Yearbook and Annual Report* (Toronto: National Sanitarium Association, 1947), Godfrey L. Gale Archives and Museum, filing cabinet 1, drawer A.

184 Godfrey L. Gale Archives and Museum, File Cabinet 5, Drawer B.

185 Jacob Imaapik to Ebba Olofsson, August 7, 2007. Personal communication by email, copied to the author.

186 Godfrey L. Gale Archives and Museum, File Cabinet 5, Drawer B.

187 J. H. Wiebe to H. N. Colburn, 8 February 1963, Godfrey L. Gale Archives and Museum. Totals for Aboriginal admissions to sanatoria in Ontario are given in a summary table for 1959 to 1962. Average length of stay is also indicated. In 1959, 350 were admitted and the average stay was 344 days. In 1960, the numbers were

259 admitted and 270 days. In 1961, it was 255 and 260. In 1962, it was 171 and 222.

188 Patient register, Godfrey L. Gale Archives and Museum.

189 C. A. Wicks to P. E. Moore, 5 February 1964, Godfrey L. Gale Archives and Museum.

190 Outpatient instructions, 1970, Godfrey L. Gale Archives and Museum.

FIVE: SEQUELAE

191 "McAndrew," *Hamilton Spectator*, clipping file, LH&A.

192 Graham Rowley to Bent Sivertz, 22 September 1953. LAC, RG 22, vol. 254, file 40-9-1, pt. 4.

193 Henry A. Larsen to L. H. Nicholson, 30 May 1953. LAC, RG 22, vol. 254, file 40-9-1.

194 A study of the careers of northerners who passed through Clearwater Lake or the Camsell would be of obvious interest in this regard. Markoosie Patsauq, who was at Clearwater, comes to mind immediately. Born 1942 and hospitalized as a child, he later went to high school in Yellowknife, became a pilot, wrote *Harpoon of the Hunter*, served on the board of Panarctic Oils and then worked in administration for the Government of Quebec.

195 There is a photograph of the two women with Hugo Ewart in the Hamilton Health Association archives, dated 1955. Both have their braids still, although Mary cut hers and dressed in fashion-conscious career-girl style during her twenties.

196 *North/Nord* 9, no. 4 (July/August 1962). As a radio announcer she received letters from listeners who recognized her voice from their days as TB patients.

197 Witaltuk trained in Hamilton, probably starting in 1954. She was certainly in Hamilton in 1955, when she translated the San's Christmas program. At that time there was as yet no syllabic typewriter: everything was hand-lettered.

198 Whitfield v. Canadian Marconi Company, [1968] S.C.R. 960.

199 "Eskimo Finds Love – and Apartheid," newspaper article, 1968, Archives of HHS & FHS, Newsclips 1936–1957, box 72.

200 Ibid.

201 Anderson's nation is imagined as "both inherently limited and sovereign." These two qualifications are of utmost importance since they imply that nations are also inherently divisible – though not inevitably so, since we can think differently and choose against this tendency – we can choose unity – and in fact, by choosing federation, the New World has distinguished itself from Europe. For an account, see James Doull, "The Philosophical Basis of Constitutional Discussion in Canada," in *Philosophy and Freedom: The Legacy of James Doull*, ed. David G. Peddle and Neil G. Robertson (Toronto: University of Toronto Press, 2003).

202 Gagné joined with Frank Vallee to translate into French *The Unjust Society*, Harold Cardinal's 1969 counterblast to the notorious Pierre Trudeau and Jean Chrétien White Paper on Indian policy, formally known as the Statement of the Government of Canada on Indian Policy, 1969.

203 *North/Nord* 6, no. 3 (July/August 1959). This article was paired with a snippet culled from remarks of Anglican Bishop Marsh, to the effect that syllabics had outlived their usefulness and should be replaced. This was a jab at the church, which Spalding thought was resisting change out of concern for the costs of reprinting its liturgical materials if syllabics were to be discontinued.

204 There may have been a deeper resistance, not to script but to an expanded presence of the written word. That is, there may have been a wish to retain the oral and the dialogical. McLuhan, following Harold Innis, asserts that "the invention of the alphabet, like the invention of the wheel, was the translation or reduction of a complex, organic interplay of spaces into a single space. The phonetic alphabet reduced the use of all the senses at once, which is oral speech, to a merely visual code. Today, such translation can be effected back and forth through a variety of spatial forms which we call the 'media of communication.' But each of these spaces has unique properties and impinges upon our other senses or spaces in unique ways" (McLuhan, 45).

205 See Robin McGrath, *Canadian Inuit Literature: The Development of a Tradition* (Ottawa: National Museums of Canada, 1984). Another approach was optical character recognition, which was used in the production of Markoosie Patsauq's *Harpoon of the Hunter*. The manuscript was written in syllabics and appeared as a magazine serial before Markoosie translated it into English and published it in book form in 1969. Library and Archives Canada holds the manuscript.

206 The act lists six principles of Inuit Qaujimajatuqangit (IQ) which are to condition the use of the authority given to the Government of Nunavut by the law, as follows:

> 27.1. (1) The following general principles and concepts of Inuit Qaujimajatuqangit apply in respect of the exercise of the powers and performance of the duties of the Languages Commissioner under sections 28 to 35 and section 37:
>
> (a) *Inuuqatigiitsiarniq* (respecting others, relationships and caring for people); (b) *Tunnganarniq* (fostering good spirit by being open, welcoming and inclusive); (c) *Pijitsirniq* (serving and providing for family or

community, or both); (d) *Aajiiqatigiinniq* (decision making through discussion and consensus); (e) *Piliriqatigiinniq* or *Ikajuqtigiinniq* (working together for a common cause); and (f) *Qanuqtuurniq* (being innovative and resourceful). ("Consolidation of Inuit Language Protection Act," 2008 S.Nu., ch. 17)

207 See David Damas, *Arctic Migrants/Arctic Villagers: The Transformation of Inuit Settlement in the Central Arctic* (Montreal: McGill-Queen's University Press, 2002). For studies of individual communities, see Louis-Jacques Dorais, *Quaqtaq: Modernity and Identity in an Inuit Community* (Toronto: University of Toronto Press, 1997) and Rhoda Innukshuk and Susan Cowan, *We Don't Live in Snow Houses Now: Reflections of Arctic Bay* (Ottawa: Canadian Arctic Producers Limited, 1976).

208 Minister's Conference on Tuberculosis, Toronto, ON, March 15–16, 1962.

209 Ibid.

210 This is not the whole story, which is complicated. See A. G. Jessamine, E. J. Hamilton and L. Eidus, "A Clinical Study of Isoniazid Inactivation," *Canadian Medical Association Journal* 89, no. 24 (December 14, 1963): 1214–17.

211 The World Health Organization's tuberculosis fact sheet 104, reviewed March 2016, indicates that "in 2014, 9.6 million people fell ill with TB and 1.5 million died from the disease," but that the "death rate dropped 47% between 1990 and 2015."

212 Isoniazid, rifampin, pyrazinamide, ethambutol and streptomycin.

213 See also Helle Møeller, "Tuberculosis and Colonialism: Current Tales about Tuberculosis and Colonialism in Nunavut," *Journal of Aboriginal Health* 6, no. 1 (January 2010): 38–48.

214 It would be helpful to know just how many tuberculous Inuit were in this kind of predicament, so as to get a notion of the scope of the problem, but Møeller does not provide numbers. Was active TB more frequent than suicide? Battery? Diabetes? HIV seropositivity? Also missing is technical detail: just what were the drugs administered, in what course and with what effects?

215 Mary Jane McCallum reviewed articles on Aboriginal health in Canadian medical journals from 1910 to 1970, mostly after 1930, and found "medical boostering," that is "medical professionals cast themselves as ardent nation-builders" assigned a "somewhat heroic, patriotic status within the medical community and in the larger Canadian community as well" (115). Also, "one cannot help but contrast the image of morally, physically and psychologically fit White health professionals with that of their patients, who, while sharing the same 'isolated' geographical space, were infantilized in the medical journals" (116).

SIX: CONCLUDING REMARKS

216 A recent brief overview of the situation is François Côté and Robert Dufresne, "The Arctic: Canada's Legal Claims," PRB 08-05E, Parliamentary Information and Research Service, Library of Parliament, October 24, 2008. http://www.lop. parl.gc.ca/content/lop/ResearchPublications/prb0805-e.pdf.

217 George S. MacCarthy and Campbell Laidlaw, Report on the Southern Half of the Eastern Arctic Patrol, September 28, 1945. LAC, RG 29, vol. 2874, file 851-1-12, pt. 1A.

218 Ibid.

219 R. C. Hastings, Report.

220 Not only by being present and hopefully loyal, but literally as an armed force. Also figuratively: in April of 1956 Ambrose Shea, a captain in the Canadian Ranger Corps "made up of white and native civilians in the outlying areas," was in Iqaluit.

> The CO of the RCAF base has very kindly found me accommodation in the officers' quarters. This morning he and his opposite number, the American CO, ganged up on me ... and suggested that the Rangers should provide a Guard of Honour for US Secretary of Defence Wilson, Hon. Ralph Campney, Minister of National Defence; Hon. C.D. Howe and other VIPs who are due to arrive tomorrow . . . With the help of Doug Wilkinson, Bob Griffiths and Sgt. Sageakdok, 14 Rangers were assembled in the townsite garage . . . It is to be a purely Eskimo show with Sageakdok as Guard Commander and Simonee as Sgt. I shall not appear at all but Bob Griffiths will stand by to provide any explanations that are needed." (Shea)

The Ranger Corps exists in all northerly parts of the country, including the main island of Newfoundland and Labrador. For an anecdotal history, see P. Whitney Lackenbauer, ed., *Canada's Rangers: Selected Stories, 1942–2012* (Kingston: Canadian Defence Academy Press, 2013).

221 See Hugh G. J. Aitken, "Defensive Expansionism: The State and Economic Growth in Canada," in Hugh G. J. Aitken, ed., *The State and Economic Growth: Papers of a Conference Held on October 11–13 under the Auspices of the Committee on Economic Growth* (New York: Social Science Research Council, 1959), 79–114.

On completion of the Erie Canal in 1825, Central Canada had been obliged to undertake a campaign of canals, harbours and railroads lasting fifty years. After Confederation the ambition to draw mid-western trade down the St. Lawrence was eclipsed by the ambition of co-ordinating the regional economies of British North America from coast to coast on a rail line. It was not until 1880 however that a proposal sufficiently un-American was put to the government and the CPR was endowed with twenty-five million dollars in cash and the same number of prairie acres to get the job rolling. From this time forward, in the words of Hugh Aitken, the responsibility for creating a national economy and the conditions in which it could survive lay with the state. Extending far beyond the basic constitutional framework of government, internal security and justice, this responsibility embraced also the construction, in partnership with private enterprise, of the east west transport system; the erection of tariff barriers behind which an industrial complex could develop; and the promotion of immigration and a flow of investment capital from Europe. The over-all objective of the policy was to make possible the maintenance of Canadian political sovereignty over the territory north of the American boundary: that is to say, to prevent absorption by the United States and to build a nation state that could guide its own economic destiny and assert its independence from both the mother country and the United States, within limits no more restrictive than those necessarily applicable to an economy dependent on staple exports for its overseas earnings. (103)

222 The information is from a summary titled "Research of Inuits," compiled on January 16, 1990, by Anne McKeage from Hamilton Health Association Annual Reports held at Archives of HHS & FHS.

223 Whether this is an unfolding of which we are becoming increasingly conscious, or an endless contest between unbalanced forces, to be concluded by divine intervention or never, remains a matter of some dispute. An alternative view is that of Ian Angus, who thinks that "if one wants to understand a country like Canada, one has to begin from the centre–periphery relation intrinsic to an empire" (*Identity and Justice*, 3). For a complete exposition see *A Border Within: National Identity, Cultural Plurality and Wilderness* (Montreal: McGill-Queens University Press, 1997) and its sequel *Identity and Justice* (Toronto: University of Toronto Press, 2008). It remains to suggest that Angus's *polarity* needs to be redoubled, to include the empire-ecumene relation that is today approaching the point of eliminating anything that has hitherto lain beyond the reach of relentlessly integrative technique. We must withdraw and allow the *okeanos* (the beyond, or wilderness) to return some way toward us, or Empire will devour the sources of its own existence.

224 This is rather contradictory, but Phillips appears to be trying not to say that natural resources will remain under federal control, since, in the event of Northern provinces being created, those provinces would inherit control of the resources.

225 Typical is a story on the troubles of Cambridge Bay by Katherine Harding in the *Globe and Mail* for January 13, 2007, with the headline "'It's just too late' in Nunavut." It was paired with another article by Alex Dobrota titled "Optimistic fresh start has gone unrealized: New government faces old problems." This was accompanied by graphed statistics for deaths by suicide, crime rates, infant mortality, et cetera. They are horrific. Four years later, in April 2011, the newspaper ran a nine-part series written by Patrick White, titled "The Trials of Nunavut: Lament for an Arctic Nation." The leader was "Crime has doubled in Nunavut since the territory was founded 12 years ago this week, raising a critical question: Is Nunavut

a failure of Canadian nation building? And if so, what must be done for history's scars to heal?"

EPILOGUE

226 In May 2007 Bob Mesher, the editor of *Makivik Magazine*, a quarterly produced in Kuujjuaq by Nunavik's development corporation, visited the monument. After brushing off some insect carapaces and clots of gossamer with a whisk made by folding a handful of grass, he wondered, being a journalist and rather persistent, whether the graves were at the monument, or elsewhere. At the cemetery office, we put this question to the man we found there. He said these graves were in two groups, near the monument. He led us back to the spot behind his truck. It took him a few minutes to find the rows of individual burial places, each marked with a brass plaque set in an earth-flush stone. While looking, he mentioned that his mother had attended the ceremony when the monument was dedicated and that she was a Mohawk from the Bay of Quinte. He pointed out to us a small repair at its base. On the evening before the dedication, the monument had been delivered in two or three granite sections to be placed on its concrete plinth. This was done by setting the base onto ice cubes and nudging it into the proper position, then caulking. As the ice melted the heavy stone settled onto the caulking. At that point however, its maker saw that it had drifted slightly off centre. While correcting this by prying with a large steel bar, he had broken out a chip. He had worked on the piece for a year. "You could see the tears standing in his eyes," the man from the cemetery told us.

227 The following January a second memorial was placed in a building within the old sanatorium precinct. This was an owl carved by Iyola Kingwatsiak of Cape Dorset, mounted on a column prepared by the maker of the Woodland monument. Two tablets are inscribed with the names of the dead.

228 Simpson, Eastern Arctic Patrol 1953.

BIBLIOGRAPHY

Alia, Valerie. *Names, Numbers, and Northern Policy: Inuit, Project Surname, and the Politics of Identity*. Halifax, NS: Fernwood Books, 1994.

"Among Those Present." *North/Nord* 9, no. 2 (March/April 1962).

Anderson, Benedict. *Imagined Communities: Reflections on the Origin and Spread of Nationalism*. Rev. ed. New York: Verso, 1991.

Anilniliak, Nancy. Personal interview with the author. Hamilton: Chedoke Hospital, July 4, 2007.

Aodla Freeman, Minnie. *Life among the Qallunaat*. Edmonton: Hurtig Publishers, 1978.

Arctic Circle. "Starvation near Piling, Foxe Basin, N.W.T." *Arctic Circular* 3, no. 3 (September 1950): 31.

Armour, Leslie. "Canadian Ways of Thinking: Logic, Society, and Canadian Philosophy." In *Alternative Frontiers: Voices from the Mountain West Canadian Studies Conference*, edited by Allen Seager. Montreal: Association for Canadian Studies, 1997.

Armstrong, A. R. "The Hamilton Health Association Laboratories 1960." Hamilton Health Association Annual Report. Hamilton: Hamilton Health Association, 1960.

Arnakak, Jay. "Use of Inuktitut in Nunavut." *Qituttugaujara* (blog), October 26, 2011. http://qituttugaujara.blogspot.ca/2011/10/use-of-inuktitut-in-nunavut.html.

Ault, Murray. "Journal of a voyage on the C.D Howe June 25–September 25, 1959." Personal journal, in its author's possession.

———. Personal interview with the author. Oshawa: Ault residence, August 25, 2006.

Bailey, S. J. "Sam Ford." *Arctic Circular* 3, no. 3 (September 1950): 36–37.

Bator, Paul Adolphus, and Andrew James Rhodes. *Within Reach of Everyone: A History of the University of Toronto School of Hygiene and the Connaught Laboratories*. Vol. 1, *1927–1955*. Ottawa: Canadian Public Health Association, 1990.

Baxter, James D. "Historical Overview of the McGill Baffin Program, 1964–1997." *International Journal of Circumpolar Health* 65, no. 1 (2006): 91–95.

Brink, George Clair. *Across the Years: Tuberculosis in Ontario*. Willowdale, ON: Ontario Tuberculosis Association, 1965.

Brown, M. Pauline. "Eastern Arctic Patrol." *Canadian Nurse* 47, no. 7 (July 1951).

Bruemmer, Fred. *Children of the North*. Montreal, QC: Optimum, 1979.

Cain, M. J. *Fodor: Language, Mind and Philosophy*. Malden, MA: Blackwell Publishers, 2002.

Caldwell, Mark. *The Last Crusade: The War on Consumption, 1862–1954*. New York: Atheneum Books, 1988.

Carpenter, Edmund. Photographs by Eberhard Otto, Fritz Spiess and Jørgen Meldgaard. *Eskimo Realities*. New York: Holt, Rinehart and Winston, 1973.

Carter, Sarah. *Lost Harvests: Prairie Indian Reserve Farmers and Government Policy*. Montreal: McGill-Queen's University Press, 1990.

Chaisson, Josephine D. *Irregular Discharges From Ontario Sanatoria: Study covering the period July 1, 1957–July 1, 1958*. Toronto: Ontario Tuberculosis Association, 1960.

Charles Camsell History Committee. *The Camsell Mosaic: The Charles Camsell Hospital, 1945–1985*. Edmonton: Charles Camsell History Committee, 1985.

Colley, Linda. *Captives: Britain, Empire and the World, 1600–1850*. New York: Pantheon Books, 2002.

Comroe, Julius H., Jr. "T.B. or Not T.B.?" Part II, The Treatment of Tuberculosis. *American Review of Respiratory Disease* 117, no. 2 (1978): 379–89.

Cowall, E. Emily S. "Puvaluqatatiluta, When We Had Tuberculosis: St. Luke's Mission Hospital and the Inuit of the Cumberland Sound Region, 1930–1972." PhD diss., McMaster University, 2012. https://macsphere.mcmaster.ca/bitstream/11375/11632/1/fulltext.pdf.

Cullen, James H., Robert K. Myers, Alvan L. Barach and George Foster Herben. "Closure of Cavities in Pulmonary Tuberculosis Produced by Immobilization of Both Lungs." *Chest* 14, no. 3 (May 1948): 345–59. http://journal.publications.chestnet.org/article.aspx?articleid=1052226.

d'Anglure, Bernard Saladin, Klaus Georg Hansen and Svend Frederiksen. "Svend Frederiksen et le chamanisme Inuit ou la circulation des noms (*atiit*), des ames (*tarniit*), des dons (*tunijjutit*) et des esprits (*tuurngait*)." *Études Inuit Studies* 21, no. 1–2 (1997): 37–73.

Delarue, Norman C. *Thoracic Surgery in Canada: A Story of People, Places, and Events: The Evolution of a Surgical Speciality.* Toronto: B.C. Decker, 1989.

De Lorimier, Alfred A., and Maxwell Dauer. "The Army Roentgen-Ray Equipment Problem." *American Journal of Roentgenology* 54, no. 6 (1945).

Department of Indian Affairs. *Annual Report of the Department of Indian Affairs for the Year Ended 31st December, 1890.* Ottawa: Queen's Printer for Canada, 1891. https://books.google.ca/books?id=qNU6AQAAIAAJ&printsec=frontcover&source=gbs_ge_summary_r&cad=0#v=onepage&q&f=false.

Dobrota, Alex. "Optimistic Fresh Start has Gone Unrealized." *Globe and Mail*, January 13, 2007. http://www.theglobeandmail.com/news/national/optimistic-fresh-start-has-gone-unrealized/article17989346/.

Dorais, Louis-Jacques. *Quaqtaq: Modernity and Identity in an Inuit Community.* Toronto: University of Toronto Press, 1997.

Dormandy, Thomas. *The White Death: A History of Tuberculosis*. New York: New York University Press, 2000.

Doull, James. "The Philosophical Basis of Constitutional Discussion in Canada." In *Philosophy and Freedom: The Legacy of James Doull*, edited by David G. Peddle and Neil G. Robertson, 392–465. Toronto: University of Toronto Press, 2003.

Drees, Laurie Meijer. *Healing Histories: Stories from Canada's Indian Hospitals*. Edmonton: University of Alberta Press, 2013.

Duffy, R. Quinn. *The Road to Nunavut: The Progress of the Eastern Arctic Inuit since the Second World War*. Kingston, ON: McGill-Queen's University Press, 1988.

Duhaime, Gérard. "La Catastrophe et l'État: Histoire Démographique et Changements Sociaux dans l'Arctique." *Études Inuit Studies* 13, no. 1 (1989): 75–114.

Eggleston, Wilfrid. *Canada at Work*. Montreal: Provincial Publishing, 1953.

Ekoomiak, Sarah, and Maureen Flynn-Burhoe. "Honouring Sarah Ekoomiak." *Speechless* (blog). Last modified October 12, 2009. https://oceanflynn.wordpress.com/honouring/honouring-sarah-ekoomiak-b-1933/.

Elliot, James. "Final Chapter Written for Inuit TB Victims." *Hamilton Spectator*, December 11, 1989.

Ellis, Frank H. *Canada's Flying Heritage*. 2nd ed. Toronto: University of Toronto Press, 1962.

"Eskimo in Print." *Time Magazine*, June 29, 1959.

Ferrier, Hilda. Personal interview with the author. Ancaster: Starbucks, March 30, 2004.

Fortuine, Robert. *"Must We All Die?": Alaska's Enduring Struggle with Tuberculosis*. Fairbanks: University of Alaska Press, 2005.

Gagné, Raymond. "In Defence of a Standard Phonemic Spelling in Roman Letters for the Canadian Eskimo Language." *Arctic* 12, no. 4 (December 1959).

———. "French Canada: The Interrelationship between Culture, Language and Personality." In *Canadian History Since Confederation: Essays and Interpretations*, edited by Bruce W. Hodgins and Robert J. Page. Georgetown, ON: Irwin-Dorsey, 1972.

———. "The Maintenance of Native Languages." In *The Languages of Canada*, edited by J. K. Chambers, 115–29. Montreal: Didier, 1979.

———. Northern News. *Arctic* 12, no. 2 (June 1959): 119–21. http://www.jstor.org/stable/40506813.

George, Jane. "Taima TB Program Kicks off this Week." *Nunatsiaq News*, April 4, 2011. http://www.nunatsiaqonline.ca/stories /article/04445_taima_tb_program_kicks_off_this_week.

Godfrey, Charles. "Taming the Gorilla: An Inquiry into the Cost of Drugs in Canada." *Literary Review of Canada* 12, no. 9 (November 2004): 14–16.

Graburn, Nelson. "Culture as Narrative." In Stern and Stevenson, *Critical Inuit Studies*, 139–54.

Granatstein, J. L. *How Britain's Weakness Forced Canada into the Arms of the United States*. Toronto: University of Toronto Press, 1989.

Granatstein, J. L., and Norman Hillmer. *For Better or for Worse: Canada and the United States to the 1990s*. Toronto: Copp Clark Pitman, 1991.

Grant, Shelagh D. "A Case of Compounded Error: The Inuit Resettlement Project, 1953, and the Government Response, 1990." *Northern Perspectives* 19, no. 1 (Spring 1991): 3–29.

Grygier, Pat Sandiford. *A Long Way from Home: The Tuberculosis Epidemic among the Inuit*. Montreal: McGill-Queen's University Press, 1994. Reprint, Montreal: McGill-Queen's University Press, 1997.

Grzybowski, S., K. Styblo and E. Dorken. "Tuberculosis in Eskimos." Supplement, *Tubercle* 57 no. S4 (December 1976): S1–S58.

Hankins, Gerald W. *Sunrise over Pangnirtung: The Story of Otto Schaefer, M.D.* Calgary: Arctic Institute of North America of the University of Calgary, 2000.

Harding, Katherine. "'It's Just Too Late' in Nunavut." *Globe and Mail,* January 13, 2007. http://www.theglobeandmail.com/news /national/its-just-too-late-in-nunavut/article17989372/.

Harper, Kenn. "Inuit Writing Systems in Nunavut." In *Nunavut: Inuit Regain Control of Their Lands and Their Lives,* edited by Jens Dahl, Jack Hicks and Peter Jull, 154–68. Copenhagen: International Work Group for Indigenous Affairs, 2000.

———. "Inuktitut Writing Systems: The Current Situation." *Inuktitut* 53 (September 1983): 36–84. https://www.itk.ca /publication/magazine/inuktitut/back-issues/inuktitut-magazine -1983-53.

———. "Mary Cousins – A Life Remembered." *Inuktitut* 103 (Summer 2007): 36–42. https://www.itk.ca/publication/magazine /inuktitut/back-issues/inuktitut-magazine-2007-103.

Harrison, Phyllis. "Eskimos in Transition." *North/Nord* (October 1962).

Hicks, F. H. "The Eastern Arctic Medical Patrol." Correspondence. *Canadian Medical Association Journal* 100, no. 11 (March 15, 1969): 537–38. http://www.ncbi.nlm.nih.gov/pmc/articles/PMC1945767/.

Hinds, Margery. *High Arctic Venture.* Toronto: Ryerson Press, 1968.

Igartua, José E. *The Other Quiet Revolution: National Identities in English Canada, 1945–71.* Vancouver: University of British Columbia Press, 2006.

Ipellie, Alootook. "Ipellie's Shadow: A Thousand-Pound Typewriter." *Nunatsiaq News,* April 26, 1996. http://www.nunatsiaqonline.ca /archives/back-issues/week/60426.html.

Irniq, Peter. "The Staying Force of Inuit Knowledge." In *A Will to Survive: Indigenous Essays on the Politics of Culture, Language, and Identity,* edited by Stephen Greymorning, 18–31. New York: McGraw-Hill, 2004.

James, Elliot. "Final Chapter Written for Inuit TB Victims." *Hamilton Spectator,* December 11, 1989.

Jeanes, C. W., O. Schaefer and L. Eidus. "Comparative Blood Levels and Metabolism of INH and an INH-Matrix Preparation in Fast and Slow Inactivators." *Canadian Medical Association Journal* 109, no. 6 (September 15, 1973): 483–87.

Jenness, Diamond. "The Economic Situation of the Eskimo." In Valentine and Vallee, *Eskimo of the Canadian Arctic*, 127–48.

Jones, David S. "The Health Care Experiments at Many Farms: The Navajo, Tuberculosis, and the Limits of Modern Medicine, 1952–1962." *Bulletin of the History of Medicine* 76, no. 4 (Winter 2002): 749–90.

Kelley, Bartram. "Helicopter Stability with Young's Lifting Rotor." *SAE Transactions* 53 (1945): 685–90.

Kordan, Bohdan S. *Enemy Aliens, Prisoners of War: Internment in Canada during the Great War*. Montreal: McGill-Queen's University Press, 2002.

Kusugak, Jose Amaujaq. "Arctic Indigenous Languages Symposium: Jose Kusugak." Arctic Indigenous Languages Symposium, Tromsø, Norway. Filmed October 20, 2008. Isuma TV, 15:37. http://www.isuma.tv/arctic-languages/arctic-indigenous-languages -symposium-jose-kusugak.

Larmour, Jean B. D. *A Matter of Life and Breath: The 75 Year History of the Saskatchewan Anti-Tuberculosis League and the Saskatchewan Lung Association: A History of the Saskatchewan Lung Association*. Saskatoon: Saskatchewan Lung Association, 1987.

Lee, Betty. *Lutiapik*. Toronto: McClelland and Stewart, 1975.

Lee, Fred. Personal interview with the author. Hamilton: office of Commissionaires Hamilton, December 12, 2005.

McKnight, Marion. "Eskimos Adjust Quickly." *Bulletin of the Canadian Tuberculosis Association*, September 1959.

Macpherson, Norman John. *Dreams & Visions: Education in the Northwest Territories from Early Days to 1984*. Edited by Roderick Duncan Macpherson. Yellowknife: Northwest Territories Education, 1991.

Marcus, Alan Rudolph. *Relocating Eden: The Image and Politics of Inuit Exile in the Canadian Arctic.* Hanover, NH: University Press of New England, 1995.

McCallum, Mary Jane. "This Last Frontier: Isolation and Aboriginal Health." *Canadian Bulletin of Medical History/Bulletin canadien d'histoire de la médecine* 22, no. 1 (2005): 103–20.

McCuaig, Katherine. *The Weariness, the Fever and the Fret: The Campaign against Tuberculosis in Canada, 1900–1950.* Montreal: McGill-Queen's University Press, 1999.

McGrath, Robin. *Canadian Inuit Literature: The Development of a Tradition.* Ottawa: National Museums of Canada, 1984.

McLuhan, Marshall. *The Gutenberg Galaxy: The Making of Typographic Man.* Toronto: University of Toronto Press, 1962.

Merridale, Catherine. *Night of Stone: Death and Memory in Twentieth-Century Russia.* New York: Viking, 2001.

Miller, F. J. W., R. M. E. Seal and Mary D. Taylor. *Tuberculosis in Children: Evolution, Control, Treatment.* London: Churchill, 1963.

Milloy, John S. *"A National Crime": The Canadian Government and the Residential School System, 1879–1986.* Winnipeg: University of Manitoba Press, 1999.

Møeller, Helle. "A Problem of the Government? Colonization and the Socio-Cultural Experience of Tuberculosis in Nunavut." M.A. thesis, University of Copenhagen, 2005.

Mortimer, Edward A., Jr. "Pertussis." In *Bacterial Infections of Humans: Epidemiology and Control,* edited by Alfred S. Evans and Philip S. Brachman, 529–41. New York: Plenum Medical, 1998.

Neuman, Kathe. Personal interview with the author. Ancaster: Neuman residence, June 25, 2004.

Niethammer, Caroline. *I'll Go and Do More: Annie Dodge Wauneka, Navajo Leader and Activist.* Lincoln: University of Nebraska Press, 2001.

Nixon, P. G. "Early Administrative Developments in Fighting Tuberculosis among Canadian Inuit: Bringing State Institutions Back In." *Northern Review* 2 (Winter 1988): 67–84.

"Nunavut health group to commemorate Inuit TB victims." *CBC News*, September 11, 2007. http://www.cbc.ca/news/canada/north/nunavut-health-group-to-commemorate-inuit-tb-victims-1.642601.

Olofsson, Ebba. "Remembrance of Illness and Recovery: Identity Changes of Inuit Men and Women Who Were Treated in Southern Hospitals in the 1950s." Presentation at the Canadian Rural Health Society and the Canadian Society for Circumpolar Health joint conference, Québec City, QC, Friday, October 28, 2005.

Owram, Doug. *The Government Generation: Canadian Intellectuals and the State, 1900–1945*. Toronto: University of Toronto Press, 1986.

Paddon, W. A. *Labrador Doctor: My Life with the Grenfell Mission*. Toronto: James Lorimer, 1989.

Padlo, Ann. "Turn of the Screw." *North/Nord* 6, no. 3 (July/August 1959): 7.

Page, Carl. *Philosophical Historicism and the Betrayal of First Philosophy*. University Park: Pennsylvania State University Press, 1995.

Pagel, Walter, F. A. H. Simmonds, Norman Macdonald and E. Nassau. *Pulmonary Tuberculosis: Bacteriology, Pathology, Diagnosis, Management, Epidemiology, and Prevention*. 4th ed. London: Oxford University Press, 1964.

Paine, Robert. "The Nursery Game: Colonizers and Colonized in the Canadian Arctic." *Études Inuit Studies* 1, no. 1 (1977): 5–32.

Palermo, Jr., Anthony. "A Legacy of Caring: The History of Picker International." *GEC Review* 10, no. 2 (1995). Accessed on January 16, 2012. http://picker-roentgen.de/picker_history_apalermo.pdf (site discontinued).

Patterson, Kevin. *Consumption*. Toronto: Vintage Canada, 2006.
———. "TB: The Patient Predator." *Mother Jones*, March/April 2003. http://www.motherjones.com/politics/2003/03/patient-predator.

Petite, Robert. "The Bell 47 Helicopter in Canada: The Early Years 1946-47." Bell 47. 2006. Accessed January 13, 2012. http://cellmath.med.utotonto.ca/B47/history/47Canada.html (site discontinued).

Pickstone, John V. *Ways of Knowing: A New History of Science, Technology, and Medicine.* Chicago: University of Chicago Press, 2001.

Phillips, R. A. J. *Canada's North.* Toronto: Macmillan of Canada, 1967.

Pryde, Duncan. *Nunaga: Ten Years of Eskimo Life.* New York: Walker, 1972.

"QTC Background Reports: Updates & Executive Summaries." Paper prepared for the Annual General Meeting of the Qikiqtani Inuit Association, Iqaluit, NU, October 21, 2009. http://www.qtcommission.com/documents/main/ QTCTestimonySummariesForQIA_AGM.pdf.

Purdy, Al. "A Sort of Human Triumph." *Imperial Oil Review* (Autumn 1999): 20–23.

Rabinowitz (née van der Woerd), Johanna. Personal interviews with the author. Hamilton, ON: Rabinowitz residence, March 25, 2004; April 7, 2004; January 20, 2005; November 16, 2005; November 30, 2005; January 18, 2006; February 22, 2006 and June 7, 2006.

Roberts, Barbara. *Whence They Came: Deportation from Canada, 1900–1935.* Ottawa: University of Ottawa Press, 1988.

Robertson, Gordon. *Memoirs of a Very Civil Servant: Mackenzie King to Pierre Trudeau.* Toronto: University of Toronto Press, 2000.

Rosenberg, Louis. *Canada's Jews: A Social and Economic Study of Jews in Canada in the 1930s.* Edited by Morton Weinfeld. Montreal: McGill-Queen's University Press, 1993.

Royal Canadian Air Force. "Operation Box Top – the Big Lift." *North/Nord* 11, no. 6 (November/December 1964): 8.

Ryan, Frank. *The Forgotten Plague: How the Battle against Tuberculosis Was Won – and Lost.* New York: Little, Brown, 1993.

Saimaiyuk, Sarah, and Simon Saimaiyuk. "Life as a TB Patient in the South." *Inuktitut* 71 (1990): 20–29. https://www.itk.ca/publication/magazine/inuktitut/back-issues/inuktitut-magazine-1990-71.

Schaefer, Otto. "Medical Observations and Problems in the Canadian Arctic." Pt 2. *Canadian Medical Association Journal* 81, no. 5 (September 1959): 386–93. http://www.ncbi.nlm.nih.gov/pmc/articles/PMC1831365/.

Schmalz, Peter S. *The Ojibwa of Southern Ontario.* Toronto: University of Toronto Press, 1991.

Selway (née Van wan Rooy), Gerda. Personal interviews with the author. Dundas, ON: February 16, 2004 and February 26, 2004.

Shea, Ambrose. "Rangers of Frobisher." *The Beaver* (Winter 1956).

Sivertz, Ben. "We Will Not Do an Article for North," *North/Nord* 9, no. 1 (January/February 1962): 25.

Smith, F. B. *The Retreat of Tuberculosis, 1850–1950.* London: Croom Helm, 1988.

Smith, Graeme. "Ship's Passage Opens Old Wounds." *Globe and Mail*, July 9, 2004. http://www.theglobeandmail.com/news/national/ships-passage-opens-old-wounds/article20433727/.

———. 2008. "Troops Goals Appear More Distant." *Globe and Mail*, December 6, 2008. http://www.theglobeandmail.com/news/national/troops-goals-appear-more-distant/article17975724/?page=all.

Spalding, Alex. *Aivilik Adventure: A Reminiscence of Two Years Spent with the Inuit of the Old Culture.* Toronto: A. Spalding, 1994.

———. "'No Frigate like a Book': Developments on the Tentative Standard Orthography for Eskimos." *North/Nord* 9, no. 2 (April 1962).

———. *North/Nord* 6, no. 3 (July/August 1959).

Stern, Pamela, and Lisa Stevenson, eds. *Critical Inuit Studies: An Anthology of Contemporary Arctic Ethnography.* Lincoln: University of Nebraska Press, 2006.

Stevenson, Alex. "The 1951 Eastern Arctic Patrol." *Arctic Circular* 5, no. 2 (February 1952): 19–20.

Tagoona, William. "The Radicals: Interview With William Tagoona." By Sydney Sackett. *Inuktitut* 90, 2001, 8–25. https://www.itk.ca/publication/magazine/inuktitut/back-issues/inuktitut-magazine-2001-90.

Tester, Frank James, and Peter Kulchyski. *Tammarniit (Mistakes): Inuit Relocation in the Eastern Arctic, 1939–63.* Vancouver: University of British Columbia Press, 1994.

Tester, Frank James, Paule McNicoll and Peter Irniq. "Writing for Our Lives: The Language of Homesickness, Self-Esteem and the Inuit TB 'Epidemic.'" *Études Inuit Studies* 25, no. 1–2 (2001): 121–40.

Thompson, Frederick R. "Combined Hip Fusion and Subtrochanteric Osteotomy Allowing Early Ambulation." *The Journal of Bone and Joint Surgery* 38, no. 1 (January 1956): 13–22.

Thompson, John Beswarick. *The More Northerly Route: A Photographic Study of the 1944 Voyage of the St. Roch through the Northwest Passage.* Ottawa: Information Canada, 1974.

Thorén, Ragnar. *Picture Atlas of the Arctic.* Amsterdam; New York: Elsevier, 1969.

Tippett, Maria. Photographs by Charles Gimpel. *Between Two Cultures: A Photographer Among the Inuit.* London: Hamish Hamilton, 1994.

"Transcript of First ITC Meeting." Inuit Tapirisat of Canada Meeting, Toronto, ON, February 18, 1971. https://www.itk.ca/about-itk/origins/transcript-first-itc-meeting.

"Trudeau and Lévesque team up for Fighting Words." *Fighting Words*, Radio-Canada CBC, recorded November 11, 1957. CBC Player, 20:51. CBC Digital Archives, accessed on April 25, 2016, http://www.cbc.ca/player/play/1801975658.

"Tuberculosis Survey: James and Hudson Bays, 1950." Northern News. *Arctic* 4, no. 2 (September 1951): 140–41. http://pubs.aina.ucalgary.ca/arctic/Arctic4-2-138.pdf.

Valentine, Victor F., and Frank G. Vallee, eds. *Eskimo of the Canadian Arctic.* Toronto: McClelland and Stewart, 1968.

Vallee, Frank G. 1968. "Differentiation Among the Eskimos in Some Canadian Arctic Settlements." In Valentine and Vallee, *Eskimo of the Canadian Arctic*, 112–26.

Vanast, Walter J. 1991. "The Death of Jennie Kanajuq: Tuberculosis, Religious Competition and Cultural Conflict in Coppermine, 1929–31." *Études Inuit Studies* 15, no. 1 (1991): 75–104.

Waller, Dulce. "Handicrafts Bring Profit to Sanatorium Patients." *Globe and Mail*, December 1, 1956.

Wenzel, George W. "Inuit Health and the Health Care System: Change and Status Quo." *Études Inuit Studies* 5, no. 1 (1981): 7–16.

Wherrett, George Jasper. *The Miracle of the Empty Beds: A History of Tuberculosis in Canada*. Toronto: University of Toronto Press, 1977.

———. "Recent Developments in Canada's Tuberculosis Services." *Canadian Journal of Public Health* 46 (March 1955): 97. Reproduced in McCuaig, 289.

White, Patrick. "The Trials of Nunavut: Lament for an Arctic Nation." *Globe and Mail*, April 1, 2011. http://www .theglobeandmail.com/news/national/nunavut/the-trials-of -nunavut-lament-for-an-arctic-nation/article547265/.

Whitfield, Terence John. "Aniapic and Me." *North/Nord* 9, no. 2 (March/April 1962).

Wicks, C. A. "Recent Trends in Treatment and in Operating Funds at Tuberculosis Hospitals in Ontario." Paper presented at the Ontario Sanatorium Financial and Statistical Association, October 1953. Godfrey L. Gale Archives and Museum, West Park Healthcare Centre, Toronto.

———. "Sanatorium Treatment of Tuberculosis Patients in Ontario." *Canadian Medical Association Journal* 67, no. 5 (November 1952): 446–450. http://www.ncbi.nlm.nih.gov/pmc/articles /PMC1822642/.

Wild, Roland. *Arctic Command: The Story of Smellie of the Nascopie*. Toronto: Ryerson Press, 1955.

Willis, John S. "Strange Night Ashore." *North/Nord* 9, no. 1 (January–February 1962).

Wilson, Paul. "Inuit TB Victims Deserve Better." *Hamilton Spectator*, August 25, 1994.

Wilson, Ralph Holland. *Chedoke: More than a Sanatorium*. Edited by Robert J. Williamson. Hamilton: Hamilton Health Sciences, Chedoke Hospital, 2006.

World Health Organization. "Tuberculosis." Fact Sheet N°104. Last modified October 2015. http://www.who.int/mediacentre /factsheets/fs104/en/.

Zarate, Gabriel. "Worst TB Outbreak Since 1999 Hits Nunavut." *Nunatsiaq News*, August 13, 2010. http://www.nunatsiaqonline.ca /stories/article/897679_worst_tb_outbreak_since_1999_hits _nunavut.

INDEX

Howard, Irene, 157–158

Hudson Bay, 30, 79, 83, 94, 210, 213, 215

Hudson's Bay Company (HBC), 25, 30, 60, 62, 92, 117, 123, 130, 153, 184, 185, 210, 213

Igloolik, NU, 29, 62, 63, 136

Indian Act, 107, 109

Indian Affairs, 23, 211

Indian and Northern Health Services, 18, 58

Indian Health Services, 35, 71, 119, 123, 126, 140, 162

infant mortality, 52, 100, 129, 130

influenza, 50, 101

Inuit: art, 152–153, 213; diet of, 47, 90, 212; Euro-Canadian descriptions of, 84–86; health, views on, 206–208; medical examinations of, 88–89, 95–102; myths, 195, 197; naming practices, 47, 96; political representation, 55–56, 214, 220–221; relocation of, 83, 233n12 (*see also* resettlement); tradition, 158–159. *See also* Nunavut; Euro-Canadians and Inuit

Inuit Broadcasting Corporation, 187

Inuit Language Commission, 195–196

Inuit Language Protection Act, 197. *See also* Official Languages Act

Inuit Qaujimajatuqangit (IQ), 249n206. *See also* Inuit Language Protection Act

Inuit Tapiriit Kanatami (ITK), 55, 96, 191, 196, 221

Inuit, with tuberculosis: 1980–2000, 203–208, 250n214; 2000–2010, 208; current numbers, 209; at the San, 35–36, 138, 140–142, 166–177, 244n139; treatments, 40–41, 116, 118, 200, 201, 204–206. *See also* Arctic medical surveys; evacuation; x-rays

Inuktitut, 46, 77, 91, 92, 97, 141, 142, 182, 189, 192–198, 222; Roman alphabetic writing, 163, 195, 196, 197, 225; syllabic writing, 30, 148, 156, 157, 159–165, 183, 193, 195, 196, 197, 225, 245n154, 246n170, 249n203

Inuktitut magazine, 91, 92, 165, 189, 191, 221, 246n173

Iqaluit, NU, 19, 38, 78, 162, 179, 183, 185, 189, 198, 204, 208, 209, 222. *See also* Frobisher Bay

Irniq, Peter, 23, 106, 125, 243n127

Irregular Discharges from Ontario Sanatoria (Chaisson), 168

isoniazid, 33, 34, 39, 40, 41, 43, 51, 52, 53, 59, 176, 202

isonicotinic acid hydrazide (INH), 16, 18, 31, 32, 34, 36, 43, 51, 57, 58, 135, 144, 147, 151, 201

Ittinuar, Peter, 183

Ivujivik, QC, 30, 103, 213

James Bay, 18, 35, 40, 89, 93, 156, 169, 173, 179, 184

Japanese-Canadians, 21, 27–28, 138

Jenness, Diamond, 21

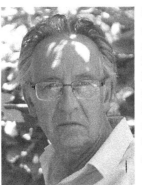

Shawn Selway's writing has appeared in literary journals and on a local civic affairs blog in Hamilton, Ontario, where he lives. He is a millwright by trade and operates a consultancy in the conservation of historic machinery. He is interested in the relation between technical and political solutions.